Telephone Triage for Oncology Nurses

Margaret Hickey, RN, MSN, MS, OCN®, CORLN, and

Susan Newton, RN, MS, AOCN®

Oncology Nursing Society
Pittsburgh, PA

ONS Publishing Division
Publisher: Leonard Mafrica, MBA, CAE
Director, Commercial Publishing/Technical Publications Editor: Barbara Sigler, RN, MNEd
Technical Publications Editor: Angela Klimaszewski, RN, MSN
Production Manager: Lisa M. George, BA
Staff Editor: Lori Wilson, BA
Graphic Designer: Dany Sjoen

Telephone Triage for Oncology Nurses

First printing, July 2004
Second printing, November 2004
Third printing, December 2005

Library of Congress Control Number: 2004109246

ISBN 1-890504-47-5

Publisher's Note

This book is published by the Oncology Nursing Society (ONS). ONS neither represents nor guarantees that the practices described herein will, if followed, ensure safe and effective patient care. The recommendations contained in this book reflect ONS's judgment regarding the state of general knowledge and practice in the field as of the date of publication. The recommendations may not be appropriate for use in all circumstances. Those who use this book should make their own determinations regarding specific safe and appropriate patient-care practices, taking into account the personnel, equipment, and practices available at the hospital or other facility at which they are located. The editors and publisher cannot be held responsible for any liability incurred as a consequence from the use or application of any of the contents of this book. Figures and tables are used as examples only. They are not meant to be all-inclusive, nor do they represent endorsement of any particular institution by ONS. Mention of specific products and opinions related to those products do not indicate or imply endorsement by ONS. The opinions and ideas expressed in this book are those of authors and are not to be construed as the opinions or recommendations of Ortho Biotech.

ONS publications are originally published in English. Permission has been granted by the ONS Board of Directors for foreign translation. (Individual tables and figures that are reprinted or adapted require additional permission from the original source.) However, because translations from English may not always be accurate or precise, ONS disclaims any responsibility for inaccuracies in words or meaning that may occur as a result of the translation. Readers relying on precise information should check the original English version.

Printed in the United States of America

Oncology Nursing Society
Integrity • Innovation • Stewardship • Advocacy • Excellence • Inclusiveness

Contributors

EDITORS

Margaret Hickey, RN, MSN, MS, OCN®, CORLN
Senior Manager, Clinical Affairs
Ortho Biotech
La Place, Louisiana

Susan Newton, RN, MS, AOCN®
Field Manager, Oncology Nursing
Ortho Biotech
Dayton, Ohio

Protocol Authors

Terri Armen, RN
Research Nurse
Sarcoma Medical Oncology
University of Texas M.D. Anderson
    Cancer Center
Houston, Texas

Linda Bracks-Madison, RN, BSN
Clinical Nurse, Outpatient
University of Texas M.D. Anderson
    Cancer Center
Houston, Texas

Jane Clark, PhD, RN, AOCN®,
    APRN-BC
Oncology Nursing Consultant
Decatur, Georgia

Denise Dearing, RN, BSN, OCN®
Oncology Nurse Information
    Specialist
American Cancer Society
Austin, Texas

Christy Erikson, RN, MSN, NP,
    AOCN®
Nurse Practitioner, Hematology/
    Oncology Clinic
Fletcher Allen Health Care
Burlington, Vermont

Karen Feldmeyer, RD, LD
Registered Licensed Dietitian
Department of Radiation Oncology
Miami Valley Hospital
Dayton, Ohio

Lisa Feldsien, RN, BSN, OCN®
Staff Nurse
Radiation Oncology Department
Western Baptist Hospital
Paducah, Kentucky

Kathy Fister, RN, OCN®
Assistant Nurse Manager, Ambula-
   tory Treatment Center
M.D. Anderson Cancer Center
   Orlando
Orlando, Florida

Patricia I. Geddie, RN, MS, AOCN®
Education Coordinator II/Specialist
M.D. Anderson Cancer Center
   Orlando
Orlando, Florida

Mary K. Hughes, MS, RN, CNS
Clinical Nurse Specialist
Psychiatry Section
Neuro-Oncology Department
University of Texas M.D. Anderson
   Cancer Center
Houston, Texas

Anne Invernale, RN, BSN
Chief Operating Officer
Empire State PolyPlants, Inc. and
   Atlantic PolyPlants, Inc.
Co-Founder, Executive Director,
   and President
Hortus Carus Foundation, Inc.
New York, New York

Nancy Lange, RN, OCN®
Weekend Telephone Triage Nurse
Cancer Care Associates
Oklahoma City, Oklahoma

Nan Lawary, RN, BSN, OCN®
Staff Nurse
Hematology/Oncology Clinic
Department of Veterans Affairs
   Medical Center
Dayton, Ohio

Lori Lindsey, RNC, FNP, OCN®
Nurse Practitioner
Texas Cancer Associates
Dallas, Texas

Victoria Wochna Loerzel, MSN,
   RN, OCN®
Project Director
Breast Cancer Survivor Study
School of Nursing
University of Central Florida
Orlando, Florida

Rita Mahaffey, RN, BSN, OCN®
Breast Care Coordinator
M.D. Anderson Cancer Center
   Orlando
Orlando, Florida

Joyce Marrs, RN, BSN, OCN®
Staff Nurse
Medical Oncology Hematology
   Associates, Inc.
Dayton, Ohio

Jackie Matthews, RN, MS, AOCN®
Oncology Clinical Nurse Specialist
Miami Valley Hospital
Dayton, Ohio

Sandra A. Mitchell, CRNP, MScN,
   AOCN®
Oncology Nurse Practitioner
National Cancer Institute
Bethesda, Maryland
Faculty Associate, School of Nursing
University of Maryland
Baltimore, Maryland

Kimberly Morrison, BSN, MN,
   AOCN®, ARNP
Oncology Nurse Practitioner
M.D. Anderson Cancer Center
   Orlando
Orlando, Florida

Mary Murphy, RN, MS, AOCN®,
  CHPN
Director of Clinical Systems/
  Hospice Clinical Nurse Specialist
Hospice of Dayton
Dayton, Ohio

Kathleen Murphy-Ende, RN, PhD,
  AOCN®
Nurse Practitioner and Clinical
  Assistant Professor
University of Wisconsin Hospitals
  and Clinics
University of Wisconsin-Madison
  School of Nursing
Madison, Wisconsin

Rae M. Norrod, MS, RN, AOCN®
Clinical Nurse Specialist
Kettering Medical Center Network
Kettering, Ohio

Ana Nunez, BSN, RN, OCN®
Staff Nurse
Sister Caritas Cancer Center
Mercy Medical Center
Springfield, Massachusetts

Carol Pilgrim, APRN, BC
Nurse Practitioner
Carle Clinic Association
Urbana, Illinois

Pat Reymann, RN, MSN, AOCN®
Oncology Consultant
Birmingham, Alabama

Victoria Wenhold Sherry, MSN,
  CRNP
Inpatient Oncology Nurse Practitioner
The Hospital of the University of
  Pennsylvania
Philadelphia, Pennsylvania

Melanie Simpson, RN, BSN, OCN®,
  CHPN
Nurse Clinician, Pain Management
  Resource Team
University of Kansas Hospital
Kansas City, Kansas

Julie Snider, RN, BSN, OCN®
Clinical Coordinator
Department of Palliative Care and
  Rehabilitation Medicine
University of Texas M.D. Anderson
  Cancer Center
Houston, Texas

Dolores Tanner, RN, OCN®
Medical Oncology Outpatient Nurse
M.D. Anderson Cancer Center
  Orlando
Orlando, Florida

Jennifer S. Webster, MN, MPH,
  APRN, BC, AOCN®
Clinical Nurse Specialist/Nurse
  Practitioner
Georgia Cancer Specialists
Atlanta, Georgia

Shirley Williams, RN, CS, AOCN®
Consultant
Port Townsend, Washington

Table of Contents

· ·

Acknowledgments ix

Introduction 1

Overview 5

Models of Telephone Triage 17

The Use of Guidelines 21

Tips on Performing Telephone Triage 25

Performing Telephone Assessments 31

Legal Concerns of Telephone Triage 37

Telephone Triage Guidelines 55
    Alopecia 57
    Alterations in Sexuality 61
    Anorexia 63
    Anxiety 67
    Ascites 71
    Bleeding 75
    Confusion 79
    Constipation 83
    Cough 87
    Deep Venous Thrombosis 89
    Depressed Mood 93
    Diarrhea 97
    Difficulty or Pain With Urination 101
    Dizziness 105
    Dysphagia 109
    Dyspnea 113
    Esophagitis 117
    Fatigue 121

TABLE OF CONTENTS

Fever With Neutropenia 125
Fever Without Neutropenia 129
Flu-Like Symptoms 133
Hand-Foot Syndrome 137
Headache 141
Hematuria 145
Hiccups 149
Lymphedema 153
Menopausal Symptoms 155
Mucositis 159
Myalgia/Arthralgia 163
Nausea and Vomiting 167
Pain 171
Paresthesia 175
Phlebitis 179
Pruritus 181
Rash 185
Seizures 189
Taste Alterations 193
Venous Access Device Problems 197
Xerostomia 201

Appendices 205
    Appendix A. Telephone Triage Nursing and
        Management Policy 207
    Appendix B. Sample Documentation Forms 212
    Appendix C. Telephone Triage Quality
        Improvement Survey 217
    Appendix D. InfuSystem Patient Education Form 218

Index 219

Acknowledgments

Special thanks to my loving husband, Jack, who entertained our three young boys while Mommy was writing. Your confidence in me is what encouraged me along.

And to my mom, Dolores Maloney, my biggest cheerleader; she'll advertise this book more than anyone by bragging to everyone she meets!

I also would like to recognize and thank Joyce Marrs, RN, BSN, OCN®, and Judy Lundgren, RN, MS, AOCN®, for their thoughtful review of this book.
—Susie Newton

This book could not have been possible without the contributions of nurses across the country who sent in telephone protocols—thank you all. A special thanks to Yvette Payne, RN, CSN, MSN, MBA, and Lisa Schulmeister, RN, MN, CS, OCN®, who reviewed the text and provided thoughtful, yet kind, feedback.

Most of all, I could not have completed this book without the encouragement, support, and even proofreading by my husband, Kenny. He always was there to encourage me as I was sequestered in my office for endless hours working on this text.
—Margie Hickey

Introduction

Margaret Hickey, RN, MSN, MS, OCN®, CORLN

Much of the care of patients with cancer has shifted from the inpatient arena to the outpatient setting in the last decade. The traditional nursing role has been challenged by this change in patient care settings. Nurses continue to be educated and cultured in the inpatient hospital setting, yet many nurses find themselves practicing in the outpatient setting. Outpatient nursing employs many of the skills learned in the inpatient setting; however, there is a shift from the nursing-based model of practice to the medical model. Nursing Spectrum, an RN-led communications company, describes the desirable skill set for ambulatory nurses, including phlebotomy, IV therapy, triage and telephone advice, teaching, communication skills, autonomy, and independence ("Careers in Nursing," n.d.).

Telephone triage and providing telephone advice is a skill set that is key to ambulatory nursing. Telephone triage and advice are new to nurses as they move on to the ambulatory setting, and overall. Regardless of the nursing specialty (e.g., pediatrics, family medicine, oncology), nurses in outpatient clinics frequently find themselves performing assessments and providing triage and advice over the telephone. Telephone calls from patients are a major component of oncology outpatient nursing practice and should be taken into consideration when budgeting for and assigning staff.

Telephone triage is a growing practice within physicians' offices as healthcare providers seek ways to identify new cost-effective strategies. Telephone call centers have been designed to match the patient's needs with the appropriate resource. Nurses provide triage and advice to callers. Patients are calling more frequently for advice and/or counseling before requesting an appointment (Wheeler & Siebelt, 1997). Telephone nursing has become an everyday function of nursing care in a variety of settings. The types of calls received and the care provided need to be individualized to the setting, the patient, and his or her problem. Mastery of telephone triage has become a difficult yet necessary skill for the outpatient nurse. Office triage nurses must be knowledgeable about the patient, including his or her current and past medical history and social situation, and experienced in the nursing specialty, with an expert knowledge base of the usual disease states or conditions and treatment regimens. The nurse must possess good interviewing skills and well-developed telephone assessment skills (Kelley & Mashburn, 1990).

Oncology nurses are especially challenged in meeting their patients' needs over the telephone. A nursing assessment of a patient with cancer can be quite complicated. The cancer, as well as side effects from treatment with surgery, radiation, chemotherapy and biotherapy, can lead to a variety of symptoms. The nurse may be taken off guard by the patient's telephone call, as it can occur at any time. The patient's chart, with a complete medical and cancer history and treatment plan, may not be available when the nurse first responds to the call. (Tip: Have the secretary/receptionist locate the chart prior to transferring the call to the triage nurse.) The complex patient assessment is made even more difficult when the assessment is performed over the telephone because the nurse is unable to directly observe or examine the patient.

Nurses are direct care providers. They are educated and practice in settings in which they use their senses when assessing and caring for patients. As nurses gain more experience, they assimilate and process information through their senses so rapidly that they often are unaware of individual thought processes. This is commonly described as "intuition" or "a gut feeling." Regardless of how the nurse defines this ability, the thorough nursing assessment, including sensory observations, allows the expert nurse to make prompt and accurate decisions. This "intuition" often is lost when the assessment is performed on the telephone because of the lack of sensory input. The nurse cannot see, touch, or smell and must rely solely on verbal and listening skills. Furthermore, the nurse may be communicating with a family member or friend who is attempting to describe the patient's complaint.

It is not surprising that telephone triage can be a daunting task for an oncology nurse unless the nurse is well prepared. A systematic process, including written protocols or guidelines, complete and concise documentation, and processes within the busy practice setting, allows the nurse to give the required time and attention to the patient's call. Preparedness requires an in-depth understanding of oncology and oncology care and excellent assessment and telephone communication skills. Oncology nurses with years of experience and skill in telephone assessment and communication may develop a "telephone intuition" that allows them to ask a few pointed questions to quickly get to the root of the problem. They are able to hone in their assessment not only with their knowledge of the specialty but also their knowledge of the patient. These nurses will listen "between the lines," focusing not only on the patient's words but also the tone of voice. The expert telephone nurse can quickly identify the patient's anxiety, pain, or other symptoms, such as shortness of breath. However, for nurses who have not yet gained these skills, few resources are available.

The goal of this book is to provide useful tips for oncology nurses as they develop telephone triage or telephone nursing practices in their clinical settings. To date, there has not been a text that addresses the special needs of patients with cancer or the special skills required by the oncology telephone triage nurse. The authors hope this book will help both expert and less-experienced nurses. The purpose of this text is to provide "how-to" tips for telephone assessment, communication, and documentation as well as for the telephone triage process, including a sample of legal concerns and models of practice. The telephone guidelines and protocols are symptom-based and were selected to address the common complaints of patients with cancer. These protocols offer basic structure to handling telephone calls in an outpatient setting while providing continuity of care for the patient with cancer.

This text is designed to be a resource for oncology nurses who are learning the telephone nursing role. However, the expert nurse will find this text a resource to be used when educating newer nurses and a guide in how to develop a formalized telephone nursing practice in the clinic. The telephone symptom-related protocols will assist the expert nurse as calls arrive with complaints he or she has not handled in the past.

The following chapters will provide tips to improve telephone communication and a systematic approach to performing a telephone nursing assessment; information on legal issues and concerns; a discussion of telephone triage practice models; and an exploration of the history of telephone triage. Symptom-focused telephone protocols or guidelines are included to direct oncology nurses in the development of guidelines in their practice settings. *It is essential that these protocols are not implemented without the review and approval of the physician(s) who manage the patients in the practice.* These telephone protocols are written to serve as a guide to oncology nurses to meet the specific needs of their patient population.

Oncology nurses from across the United States have contributed these protocols in an effort to help other oncology nurses and improve patient care. Each protocol is credited to the nurse(s) by name(s) responsible for submitting a protocol that was used, at least in part, in the development of the published protocol. Thanks to each of these nurses who were so kind to share their expertise. This text could not have been accomplished without the sharing spirit and collegiality of oncology nurses.

REFERENCES

Careers in nursing–nursing specialties: Ambulatory care nurse. (n.d.). Retrieved June 19, 2003, from http://www.nursingspectrum.com/CareersInNursing/Specialties/AMB.htm

Kelley, M., & Mashburn, J. (1990). Telephone triage in the office setting. *Journal of Nurse-Midwifery, 35,* 245–251.

Wheeler, S.Q., & Siebelt, B. (1997). Calling all nurses: How to perform telephone triage. *Nursing'97, 27*(7), 37–42.

Overview

Margaret Hickey, RN, MSN, MS, OCN®, CORLN

"Telemedicine" describes the provision of medical care across distance using electronic means. Historically, telemedicine centered on consultation or other situations in which a licensed physician is in direct contact with another licensed physician. Telenursing is a subset of telemedicine. The National Council of State Boards of Nursing (NCSBN, 1998) defined telenursing as "the practice of nursing over distance using telecommunications technology." However, unlike telemedicine, the most typical pattern of telenursing is where the nurse is in direct contact with the patient or caregiver. Telephone nursing care involves the establishment of a nurse-patient relationship and is facilitated by the nursing process. The nursing process is an interactive problem-solving process used to give organized and individualized patient care. The nursing process involves assessment with data collection, identification of the problem, planning, implementation, and evaluation.

Telephone nursing can be divided into two services: health advice and health information. Telephone triage is a means to provide health advice. The nurse addresses the caller's needs, such as symptom management, medications, or wound management, and provides specific health advice. Communication is initiated to provide triage (i.e., referral and/or recommendations to help address the caller's healthcare needs). Health information is nursing care provided to help the caller obtain information about a health issue, such as availability of health promotion programs, or community services. Communication is initiated with a focus on empowering the caller to self-manage his or her health (Association of Registered Nurses of Newfoundland and Labrador, 2002).

Nauright, Moneyham, and Williamson (1999) held two focus groups of nurses involved in telephone triage and consultation. The goals of the focus groups were to examine the evolving role of nurses in telephone triage and consultation; identify and describe issues that impact their practice; and discuss the implications of this emerging role on nursing practice, education, and research. Nurses who staffed health maintenance organization (HMO) and hospital call-in advice lines from two states were included. They were asked to describe what they did in their role as telephone triage nurses. These nurses described the three major activities of telephone triage as educating patients, advocating for patients, and connecting patients with needed resources. Note that they did not describe their role in the true sense of triage (i.e., sorting patients into urgency categories based on their injuries or symptoms) but rather as nursing care provided through a new venue—the telephone. The nurses included in these focus groups did not come from oncology offices; yet, this author would expect oncology nurses to describe their role in much the same way.

Telephone nursing has evolved over the decades. Telenursing first came onto the healthcare scene during the 1960s. During this decade and the next, telephone nurses became gatekeepers for several HMOs. Nurses screened calls hoping to eliminate unnecessary office visits and to encourage self-care at home. Telephone triage protocols and on-the-job training often were provided in this setting, where call volume was typically very high.

In the 1980s, fierce competition arose among hospitals, forcing public relations with the community to become a major marketing strategy. Healthcare marketers saw the potential for "Call a Nurse" to provide a community service while enhancing the hospital's image. These nurse call lines usually had toll-free numbers that were extensively marketed. Telenursing in these call centers provided health information rather than triage and advice. The call centers also served as a means of increasing referrals to in-house programs, services, and physicians. The nurse provided health information and assisted the patient with referrals and maneuvering through the healthcare system.

The era of managed care arrived in the 1990s. Although managed care has taken much of the blame for the problems in today's healthcare system, the concepts of care management and telephone triage emerged as a means to provide service and maximize patient access to care. Access and appropriate use of healthcare resources are two of the critical focuses inherent to managing patient care. Access to care includes not only clinic visits, diagnoses, and treatments but also advice, health information, and counseling. Telephone nursing and telephone triage have emerged as a means to provide services that use new technologies to accommodate and maximize access. Today, nurses act as gatekeepers, and they provide advice and information to educate and empower patients via telephone. Telenursing has become a common practice for nurses in today's healthcare delivery system.

Efforts of health plans to balance service quality with cost control have spurred rapid growth in telephone nursing advice services. It was during this era of managed care that the term "telephone triage" began to appear in MEDLINE indexes, providing credence to this new subspecialty.

The term "triage" is derived from the French verb *trier,* which means "to sort." "Medical triage" refers to the act of "sorting" patients into urgency categories based on their injuries or symptoms. The concept of medical triage began during World War I in France. It was designed to save the wounded and to not waste resources on the soldiers with fatal injuries. The Department of Defense and NATO (2004) defined triage as "the evaluation and classification of casualties for purposes of treatment and evacuation. It consists of the immediate sorting of patients according to type and seriousness of injury, and likelihood of survival, and the establishment of priority for treatment and evacuation to assure medical care of the greatest benefit to the largest number." More commonly today, face-to-face triage is performed not on the battlefield but in emergency departments (EDs). Triage skills and the term "triage" extend to the telephone in EDs and ambulatory clinics across the country.

EDs receive calls and visits that encompass all levels of acuity and a full spectrum of problems. Triage occurs in the ED face to face and on the telephone. Although there are similarities between the triage process occurring in a face-to-face visit in EDs and on the telephone, there are several differences. The goal of the ED triage assessment, such as the triage assessment performed on the battlefield, is to determine how quickly the patient needs to be treated by the emergency room staff. ED triage physically occurs in the direct care setting. The nurse uses the nursing process to guide the triage decisions. The nurse's assessment is aided by the ability to interview the patient and/or family member and examine the patient. The nurse is able to see, touch, listen, and smell during the examination. Additionally, in the ED setting, the nurse is able to record key physical parameters, such as temperature, pulse, respirations, and blood pressure. Telephone triage lines often are managed and staffed by ED employees and located in or near the department. Emergency nurses possess a broad knowledge base and are skilled in rapid patient assessment. They are accustomed to triaging children and adults who have a wide variety of healthcare problems and cultural differences. On the telephone, the ED nurse is challenged with making decisions regarding the patient acuity and disposition based on only the spoken word.

Telephone triage characterized the expanded role for nurses as an important tool for patient education and advocacy. Telenursing has drawn the attention of the state boards of nursing. The NCSBN (1998) addressed telephone nursing practice in a position paper, which conclusively stated that telenursing constitutes nursing practice. The argument by opponents of telenursing was that telenursing does not include hands-on care and that telephone triage nurses commonly use physician-approved protocols for reference; therefore, telenursing was, in fact, not nursing practice. Nurse practice acts in all states define nursing more broadly than hands-on care, and a consensus was reached by the boards of nursing that a nurse using the knowledge, skill, assessment, judgment, and decision making inherent in nursing education and licensure is indeed practicing nursing. The American Academy of Ambulatory Care Nursing (AAACN), the American Nurses Association (ANA), and other professional organizations have recognized the professional nurse (registered nurse) as the appropriate provider of telehealth nursing services (AAACN, 2001; ANA, 1996). The nursing process is clearly demonstrated in providing patient care over the telephone. AAACN has developed telehealth nursing practice standards (AAACN). Standard IV focuses on the use of the "Nursing Process in Telehealth Nursing Practice."

Today, telephone triage is a systematic process designed to screen the patient's symptoms for urgency and to guide the patient to the appropriate level of care in the appropriate time frame based on a verbal telephone interview alone—hearing and talking with the patient or patient surrogate. The nurse must form an estimate of the problem and identify a working diagnosis or impression. He or she then provides the patient or surrogate with direction to either seek care at an ED or clinic or remain at home. If the patient is advised that he or she does not need urgent care, clear instructions are given on how to treat and continue to monitor the problem at home, as well as when to call again or seek immediate care. The nurse also may find it necessary to make referrals to other services and community resources. The term "telephone triage" has come to encompass the broader concepts of telephone health advice. The key component of telephone triage is to triage the call. However, the nurse also provides advice, information, and patient education. The advice given may include recommendations for care to be provided at home, instructions regarding when medical help should be sought, and referral to the appropriate healthcare facility.

Much of the literature and research to date has focused on triage nursing as it is practiced in freestanding call centers or in EDs. This explains the common use of the term "telephone triage" to describe telephone nursing. Wilson and Hubert (2002) described oncology telephone triage nursing as "telephone-mediated care." The authors believed this term better described the nursing care provided by oncology nurses to patients, including advice, homecare instructions, psychosocial support, and making referrals and appointments. All of these tasks facilitate continuity of care and the nurse-patient relationship.

Telephone medicine as part of the healthcare system has been the object of study since its inception. Multiple researchers have examined the volume of patient telephone calls to physicians both during and after hours. To date, these studies have been conducted in ambulatory settings, including EDs, family practice clinics, pediatric clinics, and OB/GYN clinics. Regardless of the settings, the findings have been uncannily similar.

Researchers repeatedly have found that telephone calls account for a large volume of work for physicians and/or their staff in outpatient clinics. Telephone calls may account for 10%–26% of all patient contacts by physicians (Hannis et al., 1996; Mendenhall et al., 1978; Perkins, Gagnon, & DeGruy, 1993). Mendenhall et al. identified approximately 45% of the calls to be symptom related, and about half of these calls could be managed over the telephone. Other researchers studied after-hours calls and found that up to 99% of all pediatric population and 83% of all mixed patient population calls could be managed over the phone (Greenberg, 2000). A study by Hildebrandt and Westfall (2002) collected after-hours calls to a family practice clinic for one year. In this study, 69% of the calls were for clinical issues. Of these, 15% of the concerns were regarding medications, and 2.8% were about laboratory results. The remaining calls dealt with patient complaints or symptoms. The calls came not only from the patient (33%) but also from a family member or caregiver (31%) or from other parties, such as a nurse, pharmacist, or unidentified party (36%). Although these studies have been conducted in family practice clinics, the results are similar to the call patterns the author has experienced in the oncology setting.

Multiple researchers have examined the quality of telephone care because of the high volume of telephone medicine calls and the integral role of the telephone triage nurse in an ambulatory setting. Many of these studies, which were published around the same time period (Johnson & Johnson, 1990; Margolis et al., 1987; Sloane, Egelhoff, Curtis, McGaghie, & Evens, 1985; Wood, Littlefield, & Foulds, 1989; Yanovski, Yanovski, Malley, Brown, & Balaban, 1992), noted that when physicians performed telephone medicine, more time was spent giving instructions than listening to the patient. Overall, the conclusions from these studies were similar in that assessments were inadequate because of insufficient talk time.

Telephone communication is limited by a lack of nonverbal cues, which when combined with time pressures and abbreviated talk time create significant challenges. These are only a few of the trials and tribulations facing today's busy medical clinics. Malpractice costs are soaring. Good communication can be key in limiting malpractice cases. Negative patient outcomes combined with poor physician-patient communication are the two key ingredients for a malpractice suit. One study found that primary care physicians who never had a malpractice suit spent an average of 3.3 minutes more with their patients compared with primary care physicians who had faced a lawsuit (Cascardo, 2002). Although increased time spent with a patient on the phone or in the office is not a guarantee to preventing lawsuits, this study provides food for thought regarding a potential link between the time shared with patients and families and lawsuit prevention. As physicians and other healthcare providers struggle to manage their time providing adequate care for each patient, the load of telephone calls during and after clinic hours can be overwhelming. The time demand of telephone calls has been described in multiple studies of physician practices. Physicians have been dissatisfied with the extra time pressures associated with the volume of calls during regular clinic hours and after-hours calls (Fosarelli & Schmitt, 1987; Pitts & Whitby, 1990). It seems physicians are in a Catch-22 situation: Time spent engaged on the telephone seems to improve patient satisfaction, but time physicians spend on the telephone also distracts them from the time they are able to spend with patients in clinic, which also improves patient satisfaction.

The volume of telephone calls during clinic hours is significant; one specialty headache clinic reported three calls for every clinic hour scheduled (Loder & Geweke, 2002). As noted earlier, most of the calls are legitimate, and many of them are focused on patient clinical concerns. These calls account for repeated interruptions of the physician and pull the physician away from the time he or she is able to spend with patients who have scheduled appointments. Another reason for physician dissatisfaction is that managing patient complaints over the telephone removes the physician and staff from providing billable services to patients in the office. Fee-for-service reimbursement for telephone encounters is not available from most third-party payors. Major payors specifically exclude telephone, e-mail, and fax communications from reimbursement.

Weymier (2003) recommended that the physician limit the number of interruptions during clinic hours from patient telephone calls by delegating telephone triage to the nursing staff. A sensible rule of thumb is to delegate tasks to medical personnel with a lesser salary than physicians but with enough medical expertise to perform the work safely and effectively. Nurses are capable of providing telephone advice and triage, applying the nursing process to the patient's complaints. Not only is this solution economically wise, but telephone nursing complements nursing responsibilities as well. Communication, patient education, and patient advocacy are nurses' strengths. Pertin and Goodman (1978) compared telephone call management performed by pediatric nurse practitioners, pediatric house officers, and pediatricians examining history taking, disposition, and interview skills. The pediatric nurse practitioners outscored both house officers and pediatricians and had significantly higher scores (p < 0.001) for interviewing skills.

This match is eloquently demonstrated in oncology settings. Oncology nurses have gravitated to the role of telephone patient management in response to patients' needs rather than a planned role expansion. For the last 20 years, patients with cancer have been treated in outpatient settings with limited face-to-face contact—a drastic change from the prolonged inpatient stays of yesteryear. The patient with cancer and the family have multiple needs associated with the cancer diagnosis, treatment, and psychosocial assessment that must be addressed. Oncology telephone nursing or oncology telephone triage is not an expanded role for nurses, but rather it has become a role expectation.

Telephone nursing has been identified as a successful cost reduction strategy. Greenberg (2000) studied telephone nursing in a pediatric clinic following up on 90 phone calls to the clinic. Through surveys of the callers and the telephone nurses who handled the calls, Greenberg identified an estimated dollar savings of $2,360 for one month, with an estimated gross savings per call of $26.20. These savings were calculated from the actual dollars spent on health care less the estimated dollars that would have been spent. These estimated dollars were calculated from the healthcare expenditures that would have occurred based on the patients' and nurses' estimations if the patient had not interacted with the nurse on the telephone.

Patient satisfaction with telephone triage managed by nurses has been very good. In surveys of patients who called with clinical complaints, satisfaction with the telephone triage nurses in multiple clinical settings ranged from 87%–90% (Delichatsios, Callahan, & Charlson, 1998; Katz, Pozen, & Mushlin, 1978; Moore, Saywell, Thakker, & Jones, 2002; O'Connell, Stanley, & Malakar, 2001). Moore et al. and Greenberg (2000), in separate studies, identified the most common reason for patient dissatisfaction as the length of time it took to make contact with the nurse. Moore et al. also described a correlation between patient satisfaction and patient compliance to the instructions given. In this study, 88.2% of the patients were compliant with advice given, and the satisfied callers were four times more likely to be compliant than those who were dissatisfied with the results of their telephone call.

It is encouraging that numerous studies have found that patients are satisfied with nurse telephone triage. However, the success of telephone triage does not depend solely on patient satisfaction. It is imperative that the patient assessment is thorough and the information provided is reliable. Knowles and Cummins (1984) described the telephone calls that came to the ED as ranging from requests for information to calls concerning patient symptoms. The reasons for calls varied, with 15% of phone contacts being administrative calls (e.g., requests for laboratory results), and 36% were calls concerning routine OB/GYN, respiratory, and gastrointestinal symptoms. Requests for first aid information or regarding over-the-counter medications encompassed 25% of the calls. Forty-eight percent of calls were for minor problems, and only 1% of calls to the ED were for true emergencies.

Although a small number of the calls were emergent, most of the calls were for legitimate health problems. Nonetheless, these calls were considered to be interruptions to the more important work of direct patient care by the ED nursing staff. The advice provided was informal, given without the use of protocols and based only on experience. Interestingly, the reasons for telephone calls in this study were similar to the reasons identified by Hildebrandt and Westfall (2002) in their yearlong study of after-hours calls to a family practice clinic. The calls to the family practice clinic were for diverse clinical reasons, including requests for medication refills, for laboratory results, and to report patient-specific complaints. Although Hildebrandt and Westfall looked at family practices, and other studies examined the calls received in EDs, in the author's experience, these types of calls are no different than the sort of calls received by the oncology nurse. Although some patient calls may be urgent, where the patient needs to be seen immediately, many of the calls are for prescription refills, to check on laboratory results, or to review homecare instructions following a recent cycle of chemotherapy.

A study reported by Isaacman, Verdile, Kohen, and Verdile (1992) examined the advice ED nurses provided. A research assistant selected and telephoned 46 EDs for advice and presented a scenario that reasonably could have been interpreted as a patient experiencing myocardial ischemia. The research assistant called the ED reporting that her father was having "bad indigestion and heartburn." If any questions were asked, she described the pain as a squeezing sensation in the chest associated with nausea and sweating. Nine percent of the calls were answered and managed only by ED unit secretaries. Fifty-six percent of the respondents failed to ask the caller any questions about the patient or the chief complaint. Only four ED respondents instructed the caller to call 911 and have the patient brought to the ED. The data suggested that telephone advice given by some EDs is not standardized and may be inadequate to the point of jeopardizing the welfare of the patient. Isaacman et al. recommended a formal training program and use of guidelines or protocols addressing the most common complaints to ensure appropriate triage of calls.

The next study was completed in a setting where protocols or guidelines were available and problems still existed. Belman, Murphy, Steiner, and Kempe

(2002) studied pediatric call nurses, exploring the consistency and reliability of telephone advice provided. They studied 15 nurses and provided each one with 15 scenarios in which written guidelines were established. The reliability of the disposition was calculated, and the calls were audiotaped. The tapes were reviewed when the call nurse misinterpreted an urgent call as a non-urgent call. There was no significant difference in the time the nurses spent on the call between urgent and non-urgent complaints. Eighty-three percent of the nurses were in agreement with the information provided.

When the audiotapes were reviewed to determine the reasons that the nurses erred by misinterpreting an urgent call as a non-urgent one, two disturbing themes emerged. The first was that the nurse did not follow the protocol when assessing the patient and did not elicit the necessary information to make the correct disposition. The second reason was that the information was available for the correct disposition but ignored by the nurse. Belman et al. (2002) concluded that even when written guidelines or protocols are available, it is key to develop quality assurance processes that monitor nurses' communication skills and protocol adherence.

After reviewing the results of these studies, it is not surprising that researchers stress the importance of development of formal training in telephone management, written guidelines, and continued quality assurance to monitor this new role in nursing care. It is clear that nursing experience and observation of telephone triage are insufficient preparation. Nurses can telephone triage effectively and safely if they are well instructed, have access to high-quality protocols, and have performance evaluations monitoring the quality of the telephone communication and adherence to the protocols.

Systematic patient assessment is critical to the nurse performing telephone triage. An experienced nurse skilled in assessing patients and managing patient care may find the assessment process alien once the telephone is the only vehicle for patient management. The nurse continues to use the familiar nursing process; however, the approach to employing the process may change.

Assessment is based on the telephone interview. The nurse must identify relevant information and recognize problems even when the patient is being evasive. Information available in the chart, such as allergies, medications, and medical history, is integral in data collection. This information needs to be verified in the interview, as there may be changes since the last visit. Although the caller is the patient one-third of the time (Hildebrandt & Westfall, 2002), it is recommended that the nurse speak directly with the patient. This gives the nurse an opportunity to listen to breathing and voice cues, such as slurred speech or signs of confusion. The nurse's identification of the problem, working diagnosis, or conclusion is derived from the history, interview, and any objective symptoms.

Plan. Once the problem is identified, the urgency of the problem and the appropriate disposition is determined. The most effective decision makers consider the whole situation and not just the symptoms. Other factors such as age, gender, illness, recent treatment, and distance from care must be considered. The process needs to be interactive so the nurse can determine the patient's willingness and ability to comply with advice. For example, a nurse identifies a 32-year-old woman's complaint as severe abdominal pain requiring urgent care and recommends that the patient go to the nearest ED. The nurse failed to elicit that the woman has a three-year-old child at home, and there is no one available to care for the child. Subsequently, the patient disregards the advice.

Implementation. Once the urgency and referral are made, the nurse needs to work with the patient to set up an appointment and arrange appropriate transportation if it is necessary for the patient to receive a medical evaluation. The nurse must provide instructions to the patient, regardless if the problem requires the patient to be seen today or to monitor symptoms at home.

Evaluation. Before the call has ended, the nurse should review the plan with the patient and evaluate the caller's understanding of the instructions and the patient's intended compliance with the advice (Rutenberg, 2000). If it is deemed necessary, the nurse should schedule a follow-up call to evaluate the status of the patient.

The importance of using guidelines or protocols for telephone triage is repeatedly emphasized. Multiple authors and nursing organizations, such as the ANA and state boards of nursing, repeatedly emphasize the importance of using guidelines or protocols for telephone triage. Standard protocols provide written guidance of questions that best elicit information from patients, as well as advice and disposition instructions for the patients. This text provides examples of protocols designed to address common complaints of patients with cancer. Protocols do not stand alone; rather, they complement and support established policies and procedures.

Policies required include telephone call processing and instruction in directing patients' calls. Appropriate documentation of the calls needs to be outlined, and the authors recommend that documentation forms be developed to streamline the process and ensure that the needed information is captured. Policies and procedures need to be written to outline the actions to be taken by the nurse and physician and should include the communication process between the two. Finally, policies must ensure that patient confidentiality is maintained.

Protocols and policies improve the telephone nursing process; however, they do not guarantee quality telephone triage and improved patient outcomes. Telephone protocols are only as good as the nurse who uses them. These protocols will never replace sound clinical judgment and critical thinking skills. It is essential that while assessing a patient and the patient's situation, the nurse gathers adequate information from the patient's chart, the patient, and other resources, as needed. Telephone protocols serve as guidelines for nurses, especially less experienced oncology nurses, to aid them in the nursing process and decision making.

Telenursing has evolved over the years, and it will continue to change with the explosion of communication technology. The scope of telenursing is multifaceted, addressing triage, health advice, and information. The number of nurses practicing telenursing is increasing annually, as is the number of patients using the services available.

REFERENCES

American Academy of Ambulatory Care Nursing. (2001). *Telehealth nursing practice administration and practice standards.* Pitman, NJ: Jannetti.

American Nurses Association. (1996). *Telehealth—Issues for nursing.* ANA policy series. Retrieved January 5, 2004, from http://nursingworld.org/readroom/tele2.htm

Association of Registered Nurses of Newfoundland and Labrador. (2002, October). *Telephone nursing care: Advice and information.* Retrieved June 19, 2003, from http://www.arnn.nf.ca/links/telephone_advice_Oct_2002.htm

Belman, S., Murphy, J., Steiner, J.F., & Kempe, A. (2002). Consistency of triage decisions by call center nurses. *Ambulatory Pediatrics, 2,* 396–400.

Cascardo, D.C. (2002, November 7). Good communication practices can minimize malpractice risks. *Medscape Money & Medicine, 3*(2). Retrieved April 27, 2003, from http://www.medscape.com/viewarticle/443739

Delichatsios, H., Callahan, M., & Charlson, M. (1998). Outcomes of telephone medical care. *Journal of General Internal Medicine, 13,* 579–585.

Department of Defense & NATO. (2002). *NATO-only terms. Definition of triage.* Retrieved May 25, 2004, from http://www.dtic.mil/doctrine/jel/doddict/natoterm/t/01133.htm

Fosarelli, P., & Schmitt, B. (1987). Telephone dissatisfaction in pediatric practice: Denver and Baltimore. *Pediatrics, 80*(1), 28–31.

Greenberg, M.E. (2000). Telephone nursing: Evidence of client and organizational benefits. Nursing Economics, *18*(3), 111–123.

Hannis, M.D., Hazard, R.L., Rothschild, M., Elnicki, D.M., Keyserling, T.C., & DeVellis, R.F. (1996). Physician attitudes regarding telephone medicine. *Journal of General Internal Medicine, 11,* 678–683.

Hildebrandt, D.E., & Westfall, J.M. (2002). Reasons for after-hours calls. *Journal of Family Practice, 51,* 567–569.

Isaacman, D.J., Verdile, V.P., Kohen, F.P., & Verdile, L.A. (1992). Pediatric telephone advice in the emergency department: Results of a mock scenario. *Pediatrics, 89*(1), 35–39.

Johnson, B.E., & Johnson, C.A. (1990). Telephone medicine: A general internal medicine experience. *Journal of General Internal Medicine, 5,* 234–239.

Katz, H.P., Pozen, J., & Mushlin, A.L. (1978). Quality assessment of a telephone care system utilizing non-physician personnel. *American Journal of Public Health, 68*(1), 31–38.

Knowles, P.J., & Cummins, R.O. (1984). ED medical advice telephone calls: Who calls and why? *Journal of Emergency Nursing, 10,* 283–286.

Loder, E., & Geweke, L. (2002). Volume and nature of telephone calls in a specialty headache practice. *Headache, 42,* 883–887.

Margolis, C.F., Harrigan, J.A., Franko, A.P., Gramata, J., Margolis, J., & Ebersold, D.K. (1987). The telephone management of gastroenteritis by family medicine residents. *Family Practice Research, 6*(3), 148–157.

Mendenhall, R.C., Lloyd, J.S., Repicky, P.A., Monson, J.R., Girard, R.A., & Abrahamson, S. (1978). A national study of medical and surgical specialties. II. Description of the survey instrument. *JAMA, 240,* 1160–1168.

Moore, J.D., Saywell, R.M., Thakker, N., & Jones, T.A. (2002). An analysis of patient compliance with nurse recommendations from an after-hours call center. *American Journal of Managed Care, 8,* 343–351.

National Council of State Boards of Nursing. (1998, November 6). *Revised approved interstate compact language*. Retrieved July 5, 2003, from http://www.ncsbn.org/files/msrtf/compact9811.pdf

Nauright, L.P., Moneyham, L., & Williamson, J. (1999). Telephone triage and consultation: An emerging role for nurses. *Nursing Outlook, 47,* 219–226.

O'Connell, J.M., Stanley, J.L., & Malakar, C.L. (2001). Satisfaction and patient outcomes of a telephone-based nurse triage service. *Managed Care, 10*(7), 55–65.

Perkins, A., Gagnon, R., & DeGruy, F. (1993). A comparison of after-hours telephone calls concerning ambulatory and nursing home patients. *Journal of Family Practice, 37,* 247–250.

Pertin, E.C., & Goodman, H.C. (1978). Telephone management of acute pediatric illnesses. *New England Journal of Medicine, 298,* 130–135.

Pitts, J., & Whitby, M. (1990). Out of hours workload of a suburban general practice: deprivation or expectation. *BMJ, 300,* 1113–1115.

Rutenberg, C.D. (2000). Telephone triage: When the only thing connecting you to your patient is the telephone. *American Journal of Nursing, 100,* 77–81.

Sloane, P.D., Egelhoff, C., Curtis, P., McGaghie, W., & Evens, S. (1985). Physician decision making over the telephone. *Journal of Family Practice, 21,* 279–284.

Weymier, R.E. (2003). Ideas for optimizing your nursing staff. *Family Practice Management, 10*(2), 51–52.

Wilson, R., & Hubert, J. (2002). Resurfacing the care in nursing by telephone: Lessons from ambulatory oncology. *Nursing Outlook, 50,* 160–164.

Wood, P.R., Littlefield, J.H., & Foulds, D.M. (1989). Telephone management curriculum for pediatric interns: A controlled trial. *Pediatrics, 83,* 925–930.

Yanovski, S.Z., Yanovski, J.A., Malley, J.D., Brown, R.L., & Balaban, D.J. (1992). Telephone triage by primary care physicians. *Pediatrics, 89,* 701–706.

Models of Telephone Triage

Susan Newton, RN, MS, AOCN®

Although nurses have been utilizing the phone to assist patients for many years, very little is available in terms of specific models of care for telephone nursing care, referred to as telephone triage. Telephone triage is a component of telephone nursing care; however, when the processes involved are discussed in this manual, they are being referred to as telephone triage. The practice of telephone triage is still in its infancy stages, and this is particularly true within the field of oncology (Anastasia, 2002).

The concept of triage originated during World War I. It was used in order to not waste resources on victims with fatal injuries. The concept of using the telephone to obtain medical advice dates back to around the same time the telephone was invented (Wheeler, 1993). Health maintenance organizations (HMOs) instituted telephone advice services in the early 1970s. A hospital emergency department (ED) initiated the first 24-hour telephone advice program. Since then, telephone triage has become a sophisticated practice and common duty for nurses (Wilson & Hubert, 2002). However, the triage system utilized in an ED is quite different from what typically takes place in an oncology office or facility. Nurses performing telephone triage must be skilled in communicating critical thinking, clinical skill and expertise, patient assessment, and evaluation.

Several theories or systems for performing triage are discussed in the nursing literature. These include
- The nursing process
- Problem-oriented system
- OLD CART assessment
- A communication model
- Informal systems or procedures developed by individual institutions or practices.

THE NURSING PROCESS

This is the model that the American Academy of Ambulatory Care Nursing (AAACN) recognizes as their model of choice. The first step is assessment. The nurse should assess the entire situation, including not only what patients are saying but also how they are saying it (psychological status), how they are communicating (mental status), and what the environment is like (background noise). Let the caller explain in detail the purpose of his or her call. This is the step in which data are collected to implement the triage process (AAACN, 2001).

Diagnosing and planning is the next phase of the nursing process. This would include utilizing the appropriate guidelines and resources, including discussions with physicians and other members of the healthcare team.

Intervention or implementation follows diagnosing and planning. This includes applying actions such as teaching, coordinating resources, scheduling follow-up appointments, providing support, or any other necessary actions as it relates to using problem-solving skills to come to the correct solution for the patient.

Does the patient understand the plan that has been proposed? This is part of the final step, which is evaluation. Other questions to ask are will they comply with the plan, and are they satisfied with the resolution of their concern? Determine what type of follow-up is necessary.

PROBLEM-ORIENTED SYSTEM

In the problem-oriented system, a series of questions are asked using the alphabetical nomenclature P, Q, R, S, T, and T: the provoking factor (P), the quality (Q), the region (R), the severity (S), the time (T), and the treatment (T) for each symptom that the patient is reporting (Seidel, Ball, Dains, & Benedict, 1999). Specific assessment questions relating to each topic may be

- P (provoking factors): What makes the symptom better? What makes it worse?
- Q (quality): Use descriptive words to explain the symptom. For example, in describing pain, is it shooting? Jabbing? Cramping? Burning? Sharp? Dull? Nagging?
- R (region): Is the symptom focused in one area? Where is it located? Is it radiating to or from another region?
- S (severity): Use a 0–10 scale to have the patient rate the severity of the symptom. For example, if pain is the symptom being reported, then 0 is no pain and 10 is the worst pain the patient can imagine.
- T (time): When did the problem start? Is this the first time it has occurred? How long has it been happening?
- T (treatment): What has been done so far to treat the symptom? Has it been effective?

A system such as this makes it easy to remember what questions to ask the caller.

OLD CART ASSESSMENT

A similar assessment system is a form of patient interview using the acronym OLD CART (Seidel et al., 1999). The letters stand for the following.

- O: Onset of symptoms. When did it first occur? Have you experienced it before?
- L: Location. Where on the body is the symptom occurring?
- D: Duration. How long has the symptom been present? Does it come and go or is it constant?
- C: Characteristics. Describe what the symptom feels like.
- A: Associated factors. Are there any other signs and symptoms that occur with the problem?
- R: Relieving factors. Is there anything that makes it feel better or decreases its severity?
- T: Treatments tried. What have you tried to relieve the symptom? Has anything worked?

Similar to the problem-oriented system, this assessment helps the nurse remember what questions to ask by using the acronym "OLD CART." If this system is used, it may be helpful to post the acronym along with the questions to ask by the phone as a reminder for the triage nurse.

COMMUNICATION MODEL

Effective communication is critical in telephone triage. Proposed models of communication that can be useful in phone conversations are as follows (Wheeler, 1993).

Data collection phase: The nurse gathers data and listens while the patient states the problem. The nurse clarifies and asks open-ended questions to encourage the patient to further explain his or her symptoms.

Confirmation phase: This is when the protocol or algorithm is implemented. The nurse reiterates and states a nursing diagnosis in terms that the patient can understand. The patient confirms and redefines the symptoms if necessary.

Disposition phase: The nurse makes a disposition and gives advice. The solution is stated and explained. The patient listens and agrees to the plan. This entire process should average approximately five to eight minutes per phone call. Utilizing a communication model of practice, the nurse focuses on active listening and asking open-ended questions.

INFORMAL SYSTEMS OR PROCEDURES

Many clinics institute their own policies and procedures for telephone triage. The necessity for such policies and procedures became apparent with the creation of nurse-managed tele-help lines or medical call centers. These phone services, typically offered by hospitals, are of benefit to the entire community. Anyone can call in with his or her symptom and be given advice as to how to handle the situation (Briggs, 2002).

On an oncology-specific note, many of these services are offered by cancer centers. The center designates nursing staff members to triage the calls that are placed to the tele-help center. Such centers should operate under specific policies, procedures, and protocols. An example of a comprehensive policy for tele-help service can be found in Appendix A.

SUMMARY

Several models of telephone triage are used in practice today. The nursing process is the best documented model, as it is the one recognized by the AAACN. The problem-oriented system is less formalized. It focuses on specific questions used to assess the patients' symptoms. The OLD CART acronym is similar in that it gives the nurse a way to remember how to fully assess the patient's problem. Finally, the communication model suggests a method of collecting information in terms of phases of the communication process. It is important that each clinic or institution selects a method or model that works best and that all nurses performing telephone triage are familiar with the model being used.

REFERENCES

American Academy of Ambulatory Care Nursing. (2001). *Telehealth nursing practice core course manual.* Pitman, NJ: Jannetti.

Anastasia, P.J. (2002). Telephone triage and chemotherapy symptom management in the ambulatory care setting. *Oncology Supportive Care Quarterly, 1*(1), 40–55.

Briggs, J.K. (2002). *Telephone triage protocols for nurses.* Philadelphia: Lippincott.

Seidel, H., Ball, J., Dains, J., & Benedict, G.W. (1999*). Mosby's guide to physical examination* (4th ed.). St. Louis, MO: Mosby.

Wheeler, S.Q. (1993). *Telephone triage: Theory, practice, and protocol development.* Clifton Park, NY: Delmar.

Wilson, R., & Hubert, J. (2002). Resurfacing the care in nursing by telephone: Lessons from ambulatory oncology. *Nursing Outlook, 50,* 160–164.

The Use of Guidelines

$\bullet \bullet$

Susan Newton, RN, MS, AOCN®

Various terms are used to describe the structure for answering patient telephone calls. "Guidelines," "protocols," and "algorithms" are the most frequently used terms. Some may use these terms interchangeably; however, differences exist between each of these words.

Guidelines are what the term implies—a guide. Merriam-Webster (1995) defines a guideline as "an indication or outline of a policy or conduct." It determines a future action. In telephone nursing practice, guidelines are the most flexible. They provide a foundation for how and what the nurse should investigate about the symptom that the patient is reporting. Guidelines can be adapted to the patient's needs and individual reports.

By contrast, protocols are specific and meant to be followed exactly as written, with no deviation (Wheeler & Windt, 1993). Protocols can be helpful when the steps to be followed for a specific symptom are clear and do not require modification. For example, if a patient calls reporting painful urination and a urine culture verifies a urinary tract infection, there may be a protocol to follow to treat this symptom. Protocols can be limiting for a broad range of symptoms; therefore, they may be used only for those symptoms where it is very clear what needs to take place every time that the symptom is reported.

Finally, algorithms use a step-by-step approach to solve a particular patient problem. They assume an "if this, then that" system (Wheeler & Windt, 1993). Problems associated with the use of algorithms include the assumption that the nurse has made the correct assessment to begin the algorithm and continues to assess the situation appropriately to arrive at the next step. In addition, algorithms are written with specific directions that are not meant to be varied or altered. For the purposes of this manual, the symptoms will be addressed by the use of guidelines, which enable the most flexibility and adaptability for use in a broad range of practice settings (American Academy of Ambulatory Care Nursing [AAACN], 2001).

The Agency for Healthcare Research and Quality (AHRQ) is the federal agency responsible for enhancing the quality, appropriateness, and effectiveness of healthcare services and access to such services. In carrying out this mission, AHRQ conducts research that develops and presents evidence-based information on healthcare outcomes, quality, cost, use, and access. Included in AHRQ's legislative mandate is support of syntheses and widespread dissemination of scientific evidence, including dissemination of methods or systems for rating the strength of scientific evidence. These research findings and syntheses assist providers, clinicians, payors, patients, and policymakers in making evidence-based decisions regarding the quality and effectiveness of health care (AHRQ, 2001).

The Institute of Medicine (IOM) (www.iom.edu) and AHRQ (www.ahcpr.gov) have developed a list of criteria that guidelines should encompass to ensure quality guideline development (Hewitt & Simone, 1999). These criteria include

1. Validity: If followed, will lead to expected outcomes or results.
2. Reliability and reproducibility: If given the same scenario, another set of nurses would produce the same results.
3. Clinical applicability: Specifically states the populations to which they apply.
4. Flexibility: Identifies exceptions to the recommendations.
5. Clarity: Clear language is used, as well as defined terms, with an easy-to-follow method of presentation.

Referral to the use of a guideline can be an important component of the nurse's documentation of a patient's call. The nurse may note, "Patient called reporting xerostomia. Followed xerostomia guideline. Patient to call the office tomorrow to follow up on progress." The intervention and information needs to be clearly documented for each patient call and should be placed in the patient's chart.

When documenting a telephone patient encounter, the use of jargon and unclear abbreviations should be avoided. For example, LOC may be understood as "level of consciousness" or "laxative of choice." An approved abbreviation list may be helpful in properly communicating the situation (Seidel, Ball, Dains, & Benedict, 1999).

Appropriate personnel within the office or institution, such as the physician(s), nurses, and other parties involved, should approve guidelines. Guidelines should be updated as accepted practices change. A review of guidelines should occur at predetermined intervals, such as on an annual basis.

Some facilities have a policy that the patient's physician signs each telephone documentation form that has been completed for a patient encounter. This practice needs to be considered on an individual practice level. Some physicians may want to be informed of each patient encounter, and others may leave it up to the nurse to decide which encounters need to be reported. If the physician gave specific orders or instructions, the physician should sign off on the documentation form.

Another common practice within individual offices is to create check-off sheets out of the guidelines that are used. The guideline is typed with check boxes at the end of each step to demonstrate that the step has been completed (Anastasia, 2002). There is room to add comments for specific information about the encounter. Storage space and cost of printing are two issues to consider when evaluating the use of such forms. Online access to the checklists is an option to cut down on the storage space of printed forms.

Guidelines are an integral piece in performing telephone triage. The guidelines themselves should be evidence based and be approved by the clinicians who will use them. If advice given to a patient varies from the guideline, this variance should be documented, and appropriate clinicians should be consulted. Exactly how guidelines are used will vary from each clinic or healthcare facility; however, policies should clearly state how guidelines will be used and followed by those working in that particular practice setting.

REFERENCES

Agency for Healthcare Research and Quality. (2001, October 22). *Federal Register* (Vol. 66, No. 204). Retrieved July 30, 2003, from http://www.ahcpr.gov

American Academy of Ambulatory Care Nursing. (2001). *Telehealth nursing practice core course manual.* Pitman, NJ: Jannetti.

Anastasia, P.J. (2002). Telephone triage and chemotherapy symptom management in the ambulatory care setting. *Oncology Supportive Care Quarterly, 1*(1), 40–55.

Hewitt, M., & Simone, J.V. (1999). *Ensuring quality cancer care.* Washington, DC: National Cancer Policy Board, Institute of Medicine, and National Research Council.

Merriam-Webster. (1991). *Merriam-Webster's new collegiate dictionary* (10th ed). Springfield, MA: Author.

Seidel, H., Ball, J., Dains, J., & Benedict, G.W. (1999). *Mosby's guide to physical examination* (4th ed.). St. Louis, MO: Mosby.

Wheeler, S.Q., & Windt, J. (1993). *Telephone triage: Theory, practice and protocol development.* Clifton Park, NY: Delmar.

Tips on Performing Telephone Triage

Susan Newton, RN, MS, AOCN®

General Tips

The following tips may help the nurse to more effectively perform telephone triage.

1. Listen carefully to the caller. Do not assume that after a few sentences you are able to infer a differential diagnosis. The symptom should be heard in its entirety prior to formulating a plan of action.
2. Ask open-ended questions. This not only gives you the subjective information that you need, but it also allows you to assess the cognitive function of the person on the phone.
3. Collect enough information. The sample guidelines in this book will assist the nurse in asking the proper questions based on the symptoms the caller is reporting.
4. Talk directly to the patient whenever possible. It is more accurate to obtain information from the patient versus a family member or friend.
5. Hear all of what the person is trying to say. Do not cut him or her off from explaining the reason for the call. Questions asked by the nurse should begin after the caller has explained the reason for his or her call.
6. Keep in mind that assessing a patient over the telephone is very different from examining a patient in person. Remember to ask specific, non-leading questions. Avoid the use of "yes" or "no" questions.
7. Because you cannot visualize the symptom, have the patient help you to "see" it. For example, have the patient measure the degree of swelling or the amount of drainage on a dressing (Edwards, 1998). Also, determine if the symptom is new or worse than usual.
8. Because you cannot auscultate the patient's lungs, have the patient cough for you over the phone if the symptom involves the respiratory tract (Edwards).
9. Some patients may keep comprehensive records at home. Ask them if they have results of tests or information that you may not have access to.

10. Avoid medical terminology or jargon. Be sure that you are speaking on a level that the patient can understand.
11. Some patients or family members may be calling for reassurance. These are important calls and need to be addressed as well (American Academy of Ambulatory Care Nursing [AAACN], 2001).
12. Provide timely callbacks to the patient. You may want to establish an appointment time for a call or a best time of the day to call for routine needs (AAACN).
13. If you must put the caller on hold, ask the caller's permission to do so. In some cases, such as in an emergency, the caller may not give permission to be put on hold.
14. Do not eat, drink, or chew gum when talking on the phone. It is rude and disruptive to the caller's concentration.
15. Be sure there is a private area in which to communicate with patients on the phone. Patient confidentiality is critical. If patients in the office see and hear you discussing other patients' problems, they will be unlikely to call when they have a problem (Wheeler & Windt, 1993).
16. Document clearly the events of the telephone communication. A nurse's best defense against a malpractice claim is accurate, clear, and concise documentation (AAACN).
17. Ensure that a system is in place for evaluating the competency of each nurse who will be performing telephone triage. Reassess this competency on an annual basis (Cancer Institute of New Jersey, 2002).

TIPS FOR TELEPHONE COMMUNICATION

The telephone, although an important communication tool, limits communication significantly. Communication is the end result of the spoken word and nonverbal cues. According to the well-accepted Mehrabian Communication Model, effective communication is the result of verbal and nonverbal messages. The majority of communication, 55%, is based on nonverbal cues, such as facial expressions, gestures, and eye contact. Thirty-eight percent is based on the way in which the words are spoken, such as the tone of voice and pitch. Only the remaining 7% of what is understood is taken from the actual words that are spoken (Chapman, 2001). When a nurse assesses a patient over the telephone, effective communication is challenged. The nurse loses 55% of the message, if not more, because the nurse may not have the benefit of speaking directly to the patient. Frequently, it is not the patient who calls but rather a family member or caretaker who provides the information.

A common communication issue arises when patients use the telephone for constant interaction. Sometimes these patients are referred to as "frequent flyers." It is important to assess the reason for the constant calls to the office and intervene appropriately. Is it an education issue? Does the patient or family need emotional support? Are they in need of socialization (AAACN, 2001)? It may be helpful to set limits on how much time you will spend on the phone with the person. For example, say, "John, I have 10 minutes right now to address all of your concerns." You also may want to give the patient a specific time of day to call when you are typically less busy. Keep in mind that some patients may benefit from the services of a home health nurse or a visiting nurse if they are particularly uncertain about how to care for themselves.

INTERVIEWING SKILLS

Active listening is the key to a successful interview over the phone. The nurse is at a disadvantage on the phone because the patient's body language cannot be seen. Because of this disadvantage, the nurse must concentrate on what the patient is saying, ask pertinent questions, and resist jumping to conclusions.

The use of open-ended questions is critical when interviewing patients. When a question must be answered with more than a "yes" or "no" response, the nurse can gather more detailed information about the problem. In addition, the patient feels listened to, and trust and empathy are built between the nurse and the caller.

Encouraging the patient to share more information can help the nurse to better understand the essence of the problem. "Tell me more about the pain you are experiencing" is an example of requesting that the patient expand on the information he or she has reported.

Restating is another tool used in effective communication. The nurse repeats back to the patient what he or she heard the patient say. For example, "It sounds as if you are in a great deal of pain because you rate it as an 8 on a scale of 1–10." When using this technique of restating, the patient can recognize your desire to understand what he or she is experiencing, and the nurse can clarify information that he or she may have misunderstood.

Avoid using ambiguous words such as "often," "sometimes," "usually," and "a lot." The use of these terms may not give the nurse the precise information that is necessary. The following chart illustrates examples (AAACN, 2001).

Instead of:	Try:
"Do you experience this pain often?"	"When was the last time you experienced this pain?"
"Are you sometimes nauseated after you eat?"	"What times of day do you tend to be nauseated?"
"Is there a lot of blood present?"	"How many times have you had to change the dressing? Is it completely saturated?"

The goal is to obtain specific information about the symptom that the patient is experiencing without the use of leading questions.

It is important to recap the details of the call and to confirm the actions that will ensue as a result of the information that was gathered. Have the patient repeat the recommended intervention. Appropriate closure to the telephone call completes the encounter. To ensure that all of the patient's concerns have been addressed, the nurse should ask, "Is there anything else that I can help you with today?"

Handling Abusive Callers

If a situation arises where a patient or other caller becomes belligerent or abusive, the following steps may be taken.

1. Attempt to determine the nature of the problem.
2. Explain to the caller that you can better assist him or her if he or she is calm.
3. If the abusive behavior continues, tell the caller that you will discontinue the call if he or she continues to be abusive.
4. Prior to discontinuing the call, instruct the caller that you are hanging up. Indicate that the call can be resumed when everyone is calm and appropriate behavior is resumed.
5. Notify the attending physician of the situation.
6. Document in the medical record the nature of the call.

Privacy Issues

There should be an attempt to verify the identity of the person with whom you are speaking on the phone. There are several ways to do this. One method is to specify a password on the patient's record. The patient gives a password on the initial visit, and the password is recorded in the patient's chart. Each time a call is transferred to the office to discuss information that may be confidential, the password must be supplied. Family members and significant others who have been specified by patients as able to receive information on their behalf must be ready to supply the password before information will be given. Other methods of maintaining privacy are to have the patient supply personal information such as his or her birth date, social security number, or mother's maiden name prior to confidential information being shared.

Upon the patient's initial visit, the chart should be marked as to whether the patient allows for information to be left on an answering machine. A secondary or emergency contact number also should be listed. Messages never should be left with children or minors under the age of 18. If children consistently answer the phone and the patient is not available, the next of kin from the history record/admission form should be contacted.

Insurance companies and other providers frequently ask for confidential patient information. These requests should be submitted in writing, via fax or mail, utilizing the company's letterhead.

Not every nurse will be effective at performing telephone triage. Typically, nurses either enjoy working with patients over the phone or they do not like it at all. One has less control over a situation where a patient cannot be seen or touched.

Effective triage over the phone requires a superb communicator. The nurse not only needs to possess excellent clinical expertise but also needs to be able to listen carefully to the patient, decide what needs to be done, and carry through with the advice so that the patient is clear with the instructions. The tips listed in this chapter may be helpful; however, being a good communicator is the ultimate key to success in performing telephone triage.

REFERENCES

American Academy of Ambulatory Care Nursing. (2001). *Telehealth nursing practice core course manual*. Pitman, NJ: Jannetti.

Cancer Institute of New Jersey. (2002). *Telephone triage nursing and management policy*. New Brunswick, NJ: Author.

Chapman, A. (2001). *Mehrabian communication research*. Retrieved January 8, 2004, from http://www.businessballs.com/mehrabiancommunications.htm

Edwards, B. (1998). Seeing is believing—Picture building: A key component of telephone triage. *Journal of Clinical Nursing, 7,* 51–57.

Wheeler, S.Q., & Windt, J. (1993). *Telephone triage: Theory, practice and protocol development*. Clifton Park, NY: Delmar.

Performing Telephone Assessments

Susan Newton, RN, MS, AOCN®

It has been noted that for every patient that is seen by a physician, there are four phone calls that ensue (American Academy of Ambulatory Care Nursing [AAACN], 2001). This adds up to a large number of phone calls! It is important to educate patients about the types of problems for which they should call the office. An example of this would be giving patients who are receiving chemotherapy instructions to call the office if they have a temperature higher than 101°F. Effective use of telephone triage can increase patient compliance with their treatment plans and eliminate unnecessary visits to the clinic or emergency department (ED) and potential hospitalization.

Patients should be given a number to call to report symptoms or ask questions. They need to be informed of the process for calling the office after hours and on weekends. In addition, the nurse should clarify the types of calls that should be directed to the oncology office versus calls that should be directed to their primary care physician or other specialist.

Information needs to be collected about the patient and the symptom. Unlike ED triage nurses, oncology triage nurses are at an advantage because they already know their patients (Wilson & Hubert, 2002). Telephone calls to or from patients usually fall into one of three categories (AAACN, 2001):

1. Consultative
2. Follow-up
3. Surveillance.

Consultative telephone calls involve giving information to patients or family members regarding lab results or results from procedures or scans. Included in these calls are the action plan, or what needs to take place as a result of the information given. Keep in mind all Health Insurance Portability and Accountability Act regulations when giving this type of information. Patients must give permission for family members to receive information about them and should specify their names. This should be recorded in the patient's chart.

The nurse usually initiates *follow-up* calls to assess the patient's progress or status. It may be performed after a test or procedure, a surgical operation, or the first course of chemotherapy that the patient receives. Follow-up calls also can be made to check progress or effectiveness of previous interventions.

Surveillance involves a review of the patient's status. This is where the majority of phone calls are received. A patient or family member is calling to report a particular symptom that the patient is experiencing.

It is important to note that licensed professional nurses should perform telephone assessments. The term "licensed nurse" is used, rather than "RN," because of the large number of licensed practical nurses and licensed vocational nurses employed in outpatient physician offices. However, both the AAACN and the American Nurses Association recommend that a registered professional nurse perform telehealth nursing services. This is discussed in more detail in the legal concerns chapter of this book.

Ideally, outpatient oncology offices that see a large number of patients with cancer should employ a nurse to primarily manage telephone calls from patients. If the volume of phone calls each day does not keep a full-time nurse consistently answering and triaging calls, this nurse could do other duties in addition to answering phone calls. These duties may include teaching patients who are in the clinic, giving injections, reviewing lab results and radiology reports, and perhaps mixing chemotherapy. The volume of phone calls to triage in some settings or offices may be high enough to justify more than one triage nurse.

If there is a full-time position for a nurse to perform telephone triage, this does not mean that the same nurse must be responsible for this activity every day. This duty often is rotated among each of the RNs employed by the clinic. There are pros and cons to the way this duty is assigned. There may be offices in which none of the nurses wish to be the phone nurse every day; however, they may enjoy the change of pace that this role offers one day each week. In other practices, a nurse may be pregnant or breast feeding and may not wish to work in the chemotherapy area (Occupational Safety and Health Administration, 1995). In this case, telephone triage offers a safer alternative. Still other offices may have a nurse who enjoys the consistency of performing telephone triage every day of the week. The highest patient satisfaction is reported in the situation where the same nurse is triaging calls each day.

Clerical employees usually are the first to answer a phone in an outpatient office. These personnel have minimal if any medical expertise and therefore should refrain from giving any advice over the phone. In the rare circumstance that the clerical employee has a medical background, this person is not being utilized in such a capacity and should refrain from giving advice over the telephone. For example, a receptionist who is trained as a medical assistant must only perform receptionist duties.

To streamline the large number of phone calls that are made to an outpatient oncology office, a clerical employee may screen the calls. When a patient or family member is calling with a particular symptom to report, the clerical employee should record general information such as

• Date and time the call is received

- Whether the call is an emergency and needs assistance as soon as possible or is non-urgent
- Name of the patient
- Name of the caller and relationship to the patient
- Phone number where the call should be returned and how long the caller will be at this number (making a note if it is a cellular phone number because disconnections can occur frequently).
- Patient's physician
- Patient's diagnosis
- Reason for the call (using the caller's own words).

Having a standard triage form on which to record information is helpful. See examples of telephone documentation forms in Appendix B. Clerical employees should be cognizant of the time frames that collecting this information entails. It is recommended that the first person the patient speaks to informs him or her of the approximate time that he or she can expect a return call. Patient satisfaction often is improved by providing a realistic time frame for when the patient can expect a return call.

The triage form, along with the patient's chart, should be taken to the triage nurse. If electronic charts are used in the office, the triage nurse should have access to a phone and a computer to access patient information. Easy access to the patient's chart is imperative because the nurse may not know the particular patient who is calling.

The triage nurse should review the information sheet and triage the call in order of priority to other calls. For example, a patient calling for a prescription refill would be lower on the triage priority list than a patient calling about sudden severe pain. Such a complaint would necessitate an immediate return phone call. The process of triaging calls is a continuous one. The nurse should review each call that comes in or each chart that presents.

PROCESS OF ASSESSMENT

A variety of procedures are used in an outpatient office to triage received phone calls. A few of the most common procedures are explained here.

1. If a clerical employee is taking the initial information
   a. Clerical person receives the call and takes general information from the patient.
   b. Clerical person delivers the general information sheet and the chart (if necessary) to the triage nurse.
   c. Triage nurse prioritizes the call according to the patient's reported symptoms.
   d. Triage nurse returns calls according to highest priority symptom.
2. If an answering device records all incoming calls
   a. There should be a prompt stating that if it is a medical emergency to call 911.

b. There should be a prompt that the patient can choose in order to talk to a person in the office.

c. A system should be in place where the calls are directed to leaving a message for (1) questions regarding appointment times or scheduling, (2) prescription refills, (3) lab and radiology results, or (4) a nurse to call back.

3. If an answering machine answers and calls are screened according to physician

   a. The nurse working with that particular physician returns all of the patient calls.

   b. The nurse should periodically listen to messages left throughout the day.

   c. The same prioritization occurs as in earlier processes.

   It is important to note that although it is common to have a telephone answering device screen and direct calls, it is vital that the caller hear information as to what to do in case of an emergency. In addition, there should be an option to speak to someone in the office if the reason for their call does not fit into one of the listed prompts.

4. If there is no designated triage nurse

   a. The clerical person should record the initial information and take it to a designated nursing area. It should be left in a visible area, restricted from other patients' viewing. The nurses should be notified that a chart has been left and the patient requires a return call.

   b. Ideally, the nurse who administered the patient's chemotherapy or the nurse with whom the patient has had the most contact should return the patient's call.

   c. It may be helpful to designate a specific time of day for non-urgent phone calls to be returned (e.g., 2–4 pm).

The next step in the process is for the nurse to return the patient's call. In some instances, there may be a direct phone line to reach the nurse. This makes it slightly more difficult to properly triage the order of calls (because the nurse is taking them as they come in); however, it eliminates the time it takes for the clerical person to document a summary of the problem and deliver the chart and the initial assessment form to the nurse.

The nurse should utilize one of the assessment methods described earlier in "Models of Telephone Triage." When the symptom has been adequately assessed, the nurse describes the appropriate recommendation to the patient. The nurse must assess the patient's understanding of the intervention. It should be documented on the triage form that the patient verbalizes understanding of the information provided.

On average, how long should it take to address a patient's symptom over the phone? Between 3 and 10 minutes is the average range. If it takes more than 10 minutes to address the patient's problem, he or she probably needs to be seen in person. If it takes less than three minutes to assess the patient's issue, the nurse probably has not thoroughly assessed the problem. Jumping to a conclusion about the patient's problem before adequately assessing the situation, in essence, stereotypes the caller and can lead to an inaccurate nursing diagnosis (Anastasia & Blevins, 1997).

Many patients will require a follow-up phone call to assess the effectiveness of the intervention. In order to streamline the process and because of the high volume of calls received each day, it may be beneficial to request the patient to call the office back within 24–48 hours to give an update on his or her condition.

What should the nurse do if the patient refuses to follow the advice or instructions that are offered? One method of preventing this occurrence is to obtain the patient's agreement during the conversation. Statements such as "How does that sound?" involve the patient in the decision-making process. In addition, the nurse should determine the reason for the patient's noncompliance. For example, if the patient is instructed to go to the ED and the patient refuses, ask why. If it is because she has three small children at home with no assistance, the nurse can help her to problem solve.

If the patient refuses to follow the nurse's advice, despite an open, collaborative conversation, the nurse has a responsibility to communicate potential consequences that may occur. For example, a patient calls to report a temperature of 102°F, is unable to eat or drink, and received chemotherapy 10 days ago. The protocol may involve instructing the patient to go to the ED for evaluation. If the patient refuses to go to the ED, ask, "What would you prefer to do?" Also, the patient should be informed of the consequences of this refusal or noncompliance. In this example, the nurse's response may be, "You may have an infection that your body is unable to fight due to a low white blood cell count from your chemotherapy. If it is not treated, you could become sicker and could possibly die from an overwhelming infection." If the patient still refuses, appropriate communication to the physician in charge is in order, the conversation should be clearly documented, and a follow-up call should be placed to the patient. Every effort should be made to facilitate compliance of the patient (Wheeler & Windt, 1993).

REFERENCES

American Academy of Ambulatory Care Nursing. (2001). *Telehealth nursing practice core course manual.* Pitman, NJ: Jannetti.

Anastasia, P.J., & Blevins, M.C. (1997). Outpatient chemotherapy: Telephone triage for symptom management. *Oncology Nursing Forum, 20*(Suppl. 1), 14–22.

Occupational Safety and Health Administration. (1995). *Controlling occupational exposure to hazardous drugs.* Washington, DC: Author.

Wheeler, S.Q., & Windt, J. (1993). *Telephone triage: Theory, practice, and protocol development.* Clifton Park, NY: Delmar.

Wilson, R., & Hubert, J. (2002). Resurfacing the care in nursing by telephone: Lessons from ambulatory oncology. *Nursing Outlook, 50,* 160–164.

Legal Concerns of Telephone Triage

Margaret Hickey, RN, MSN, MS, OCN®, CORLN

Laws vary from state to state, and this section discusses general legal issues related to telephone nursing. It cannot address all questions regarding the legalities of telephone nursing practice. Nurses should consult their state board of nursing and their institution's legal counsel for specific questions.

STANDARDS OF CARE

Nursing standards can be defined as a written value statement defining a level of performance or a set of conditions determined to be acceptable by some authority (Marker-Smith, 1988). Nursing standards determine expectations for nursing performance. By defining telephone nursing practice standards, the responsibilities and accountabilities of the clinical practitioner and administrators responsible for providing telephone care are clearly defined. Established standards provide guidelines to practitioners, help to define nursing practice, and can assist in removing barriers. Standards should be reflected in every telephone delivery model. Standards can be found in a variety of formats, including policies, job descriptions, performance standards, procedures, protocols, guidelines, and written standards of care developed specifically for each center.

Six types of standards include the following (Dernovsek, Espensen, & Massengale, 2001).
- **Personal standards** include the actions and decisions of a reasonable ordinary person based on community beliefs, morality, and ethics.
- **Legal standards** include applicable state and federal laws. Each state has a board of nursing that defines the nurse's scope of practice within that state. The telephone can provide an avenue to easily cross over state lines. The nurse may not only be required to hold a nursing license in the state where he or she is physically located but also may need a license from the state in which the patient resides. Nurses must be aware of current and any new state or federal laws that address emerging concerns regarding telemedicine.

- **Professional standards** from professional organizations address telephone triage, telenursing, and telemedicine. Professional organizations that have issued statements or guidelines addressing telephone triage include the American Academy of Ambulatory Care Nursing (AAACN), American Association of Office Nurses (AAON), American Nurses Association (ANA), and Emergency Nurses Association (ENA). In some cases, these statements may overlap or contradict. The American College of Emergency Physicians issued a policy statement in July 2000 that recommended that emergency departments (EDs) should not attempt medical assessment or management by telephone (American College of Emergency Physicians, 2000). ENA's position statement, revised and approved in December 2001, recognized that sophisticated telephone triage programs provide quality healthcare assessment opportunities that enhance quality health care within a community. ENA (2001) outlined the essential qualities of a telephone advice program and stated if a telephone triage program is not in place, no advice should be given over the telephone. The emergency nurse should inform the person that the problem cannot be diagnosed over the phone, and the patient should either see or confer with a healthcare provider or come to the ED. AAACN (2001a, 2001b) published practice standards for telehealth nursing to help refine and enhance telehealth nursing practice.
- **Regulatory standards** are developed by agencies and organizations charged with reviewing and maintaining healthcare systems. These standards are created by local and state health departments, the Joint Commission on Accreditation of Healthcare Organizations (JCAHO), Occupational Safety and Health Administration (OSHA), Americans with Disabilities Act (ADA), and National Committee for Quality Assurance (NCQA), among others. Many of the standards written affect telenursing even when it is not directly stated.
- **Structural standards** reflect the conditions, equipment, and materials needed to reliably operate a call center. Written policies should be developed to outline the manner in which wait times, follow-up calls, and calls-in-a-queue are managed.
- **Process standards** define how the nurse will provide care and specify the type or quality of care. Process standards can be reflected in policies and procedures that outline the requirements for the nurse's knowledge, skills, behavior, and actions. Written protocols or guidelines serve to outline the process a nurse should take in response to a caller's symptom or complaint.

NURSING PRACTICE ISSUES

Role of State Boards of Nursing

The scope of healthcare professional practice is determined by state nursing practice acts, state medical boards, and other professional organizations that provide guidelines for appropriate roles of physicians and nurses.

The first step in addressing nursing practice concerns about telephone nursing and telephone triage is to address if this practice constitutes nursing care. The National Council of State Boards of Nursing (NCSBN) (1998) provided the answer with a resounding "yes." The delivery of nursing services by telephone constitutes the practice of nursing. In this position statement, telenursing was defined as the practice of nursing over distance using telecommunications technology. Nursing practice was described as going beyond hands-on care. NCSBN stated that when a nurse uses the knowledge, skill, assessment, judgment, and decision making fundamental to nursing education and licensure, then, indeed, the nurse is practicing nursing (NCSBN, 1998). The NCSBN recognizes telephone triage as nursing practice; therefore, boards of nursing regulate telephone nursing practice. Telephone nursing care is a legitimate means of nursing practice and brings forward new situations and challenges to the boards of nursing and nurse regulators. As stated by the NCSBN in their position statement, "Telecommunications is advancing at such a rapid rate that its application to health care delivery and nursing practice will continue to emerge and evolve" (NCSBN, 1997, p. 3). Likewise, the challenges and regulations related to this practice also will continue to emerge and evolve.

One of the challenges NCSBN and individual state boards of nursing are addressing is that the telephone often breaches distance and can easily link a nurse in one state with a patient in another state. Licensure and the state-based regulatory system in the United States were established with the Tenth Amendment to the United States Constitution, the states' rights amendment. This principle facilitated state development of the regulatory system to protect the public in each state. Each state has established legislation authorizing nursing practice within the geographical boundaries of the state issuing the license. States do not have the ability to grant a nurse authority to practice in other states. It is unclear if the care occurs at the location of the patient or the location of the healthcare provider (Hutcherson & Williamson, 1999). When the nurse provides telephone triage and advice to out-of-state patients, in what state is the nurse required to have a license—in the state the nurse resides or the state the patient resides? NCSBN has identified a potential resolution for this problem related to telephone nursing and other nursing practices that are blurring the state boundaries through technology. NCSBN (1998) has developed a mutual recognition model and interstate compact, which is a mechanism to implement mutual recognition of nurse licensure among states that sign onto the compact. States that approve the compact agree to allow a nurse to hold one license in the state where the nurse resides. The nurse can practice in other states covered by the compact using physical or electronic methods subject to each state's practice laws and regulations. The nurse must meet the home state qualifications for licensure and comply with all current laws. As of April 2003, 20 states have enacted the RN and licensed practical nurse (LPN)/licensed vocational nurse (LVN) Nurse Licensure Compact (see Table 1); however, five of these states have

Table 1. Nurse Licensure Compact		
States that have implemented the Nurse Licensure Compact		
State		Implementation Date
Arizona		7/1/2002
Arkansas		7/1/2000
Delaware		7/1/2000
Idaho		7/1/2001
Iowa		7/1/2000
Maine		7/1/2001
Maryland		7/1/1999
Mississippi		7/1/2001
Nebraska		1/1/2001
North Carolina		7/1/2000
South Dakota		1/1/2001
Tennessee		7/1/2003
Texas		1/1/2000
Utah		1/1/2000
Wisconsin		1/1/2000
States that have enacted the Nurse Licensure Compact with pending implementation		
State	Status	Implementation Date
Indiana	Signed by governor	TBD
New Jersey	Signed by governor	TBD
North Dakota	Signed by governor	1/1/2004
New Mexico	Signed by governor	1/1/2004
Virginia	Signed by governor	1/1/2005
TBD = To be decided *Note.* Based on information from National Council of State Boards of Nursing, 2003.		

not yet implemented the compact. NCSBN keeps an up-to-date list of states that have enacted and implemented the compact on their Web site (www .ncsbn.org).

Despite this effort, until all 50 states join the compact, variations in state nurse practice acts continue to carry challenges. For the sake of example only, the position statements of three state boards of nursing are addressed in this section—Arkansas, California, and Nevada.

The ever-evolving practice of telephone nursing is reflected in the position statements written by the Arkansas State Board of Nursing (2000). Arkansas first issued a telenursing position statement in November 1997, which was revised in September 1998. An additional position statement was developed and approved in November 2000. In this position statement, the Arkansas Board of Nursing clearly describes when a professional nurse (RN) may practice telenursing. These include

1. The professional nurse has an established relationship with the client and appropriate documentation.
2. Licensed physician and nurse must approve protocols annually.
3. Protocol clearly outlines basic information that must be documented.
4. A deviation from a protocol requires an order from the practitioner and is documented.
5. Protocols shall not include prescription drugs.
6. The professional nurse is required to follow the Arkansas Position Statement 98-6 Decision Making Model.

This position statement does not directly address crossing state borders, although the first statement requires an established relationship with the patient. In the case of the oncology nurse responding to calls in the oncology clinic, the patient should have at the least been examined in that clinic (Arkansas State Board of Nursing).

The California State Board of Nursing (2001) has stated that a California RN license is required for in-state or out-of-state RNs to perform telephone medical advice services to California addresses. This statement followed enactment of a California law in January 2000 titled "Telephone Medical Advice Services." The definition provided by the California State Board of Nursing statement is that "telephone medical advice means a telephonic communication between a patient and a healthcare professional, wherein the healthcare professional's primary function is to provide the patient a telephonic response to the patient's questions regarding his or her or a family member's medical care or treatment" (California State Board of Nursing).

The Nevada State Board of Nursing (2002) has established the following practice guidelines.

1. Only registered nurses, currently licensed in the state of Nevada, may practice telenursing in relation to patients in Nevada.
2. The nurse practicing telenursing must identify himself by name and title and state of licensure.
3. After completion of a nursing assessment of the patient, the nurse practicing telenursing may provide advice based on the use of written physician protocols (which may include over-the-counter medications), published reference guides, or software protocols approved by the medical staff.
4. All telenursing interactions, including, but not limited to, the collection of demographic data, health history, assessment of chief complaint, protocols followed, referrals, and follow-ups, must be recorded.

As clearly seen in the practice decisions by these three states, the issue of telephone nursing is being addressed on a state-by-state basis. Not only are some of the boards of nursing defining the scope of practice to include state licensure issues when the caller and nurse reside in different states, they also are defining what constitutes appropriate telenursing interactions. It is imperative that every nurse practicing telephone triage or telephone nursing review the decisions and regulations outlined by their state board of nursing and stay abreast of the continued changes to regulations in this ever-evolving nursing practice.

Scope of Practice

Defining the scope of nursing practice is the role of individual state boards of nursing. It is important for the nurse to be familiar with his or her home state's nurse practice act. The nurse practice act is dynamic, as the boards of nursing address issues in this healthcare environment, including the evolution of telephone nursing or triage. It is key for nurses, regardless of the state in which they are licensed, to avoid practicing medicine by diagnosing patients or prescribing treatment. The difference between a medical and nursing diagnosis is a point of law in the state of Pennsylvania. Pennsylvania statute defines a nursing diagnosis as the "identification of and discrimination between physical and psychosocial signs and symptoms essential to effective execution and management of the nursing regimen" (Kabala, 1998, p. 2). The statute does not define a medical diagnosis, but the *Merriam-Webster Medical Dictionary* (2003) defines "diagnosis" as the identification of a disease based on its signs and symptoms.

It is within the nursing scope of practice for professional nurses* to independently perform telephone assessments, apply clinical judgment, and use decision-making skills in establishing nursing diagnoses and performing telephone triage. Additionally, they can educate patients, analyze outcomes, and coordinate patient care. Telephone triage must be limited to assessing symptoms and offering information related to the symptoms.

The nurse needs to use care and follow policies, procedures, and professional standards. These standards should outline when the physician or another provider must be consulted to assist in handling the call or responding to the caller's concerns. The nurse may vary from the provided guidelines only when acting directly under the supervision of physicians. If the physician is not directly overseeing the interaction, the nurse is limited to employing the nursing process.

The nursing process used during telephone triage is the same nursing process the nurse employs when providing direct patient care. The steps include **assessment:** appropriate assessing, prioritizing, and initiating the triage process, including an often complex telephone interview; **planning:** choosing appropriate guidelines, following them correctly, and collaborating with the patient and other healthcare providers while referencing resources used; **implementation:** effectively solving problems and intervening, which includes appropriate disposition of care, teaching, counseling, coordinating resources, and facilitating follow-up care; and **evaluating:** documenting the interaction thoroughly, communicating with others, and analyzing outcomes.

---

*Each state board may have varying statements on nursing practice, and the professional nurse should always defer to his or her licensing State Board of Nursing.

Professional nurses (RNs) must be aware that their license may enable them to be used as supervisors of LPNs/LVNs or assistive personnel (AP). This is of particular concern in telephone triage. As clearly stated by the Nevada Board of Nursing (2002) and other regulatory bodies, telephone nursing is a function of professional nurses. In informal call practices, such as in a physician's office, AP may have years of experience in obtaining medical information from patients or dispensing advice on a physician's behalf under the supervision and direction of the physician. In some circumstances, when an RN supervises an AP, the AP is acting under the nurse's license. In these circumstances, the RN would be violating the nurse practice act if telephone advice were delegated to AP or LPNs/LVNs, particularly in states such as Arkansas, California, Nevada, and others that identify telephone triage as a function of a professional nurse. Personnel such as medical assistants and receptionists can gather basic information only; they cannot assess, triage, or make independent decisions on care or disposition. LPNs/LVNs cannot independently assess and triage; however, they can collect general information about the patient and present those data to the RN or physician for analysis or triaging. They also cannot independently educate patients, but they can provide general information as directed by the professional nurse or physician.

A professional nurse should be wary of situations when physicians ask them to exceed the limits of a state nurse practice act by asking the professional nurse to independently provide treatment information. The nurse should provide treatment information only under specific direction of the physician and approved guidelines. It is helpful to develop job descriptions that clearly outline the roles of RNs, LPNs, and AP in relation to managing patient calls. Job descriptions should accurately reflect the scope of practice, including minimum qualifications to perform telephone triage (such as professional nurse with three years of experience), accountability for outcomes, and how the outcomes will be measured.

TELEPHONE TRIAGE LIABILITY

Every time a nurse picks up the telephone, a relationship is created with the caller. This relationship holds risks for three reasons. The first risk is that the nurse is expected to maintain the same level of care provided in face-to-face nursing. This presents particular challenges, as the nurse must assess symptoms and offer advice without ever examining the patient. He or she may have limited information available in the medical chart and must rely on the caller's cooperation to monitor compliance and follow-up care. Second, the nurse must operate in a work setting, in multiple working conditions, with varied levels of awareness of professional standards among employers. The nurse is responsible to stay informed and potentially to educate his or her employer about current standards, legal risks, and new information regarding laws and licensure.

What Constitutes Liability?

"Liability" is used to describe responsibility for duties that an individual or organization is legally bound to fulfill. Nurses or healthcare organizations can be found negligent in performing duties and held responsible or "liable" for their actions. Any individual who alleges negligence must prove that the accused failed to act reasonably when they had the duty to do so and that the failure resulted in an injury that can be related to that breach of duty. Malpractice is negligence committed by a professional in the performance of professional duties (*Merriam-Webster's Medical Dictionary*, 2003).

Four elements that must be satisfied in order to prove negligence (Dernovsek et al., 2001).

1. The nurse had a duty to provide care to the patient following an accepted standard of care.
2. The nurse failed to adhere to this standard of care.
3. The nurse's failure to adhere to the standard of care was the cause of the patient's injuries.
4. The patient suffered some type of hurt or injury that resulted from the nurse's negligent actions.

AAACN (2001b) established in their course on telephone triage that once the call is answered, the nurse has a duty to provide care. The standard of care that the nurse must adhere to is the level of care that would be given by a reasonable, prudent nurse under the same or similar circumstances. It is important that nurses stay abreast of standards in the nursing literature (some have been mentioned earlier in this chapter). In addition to the published standards a nurse can be held to, unpublished standards based on the testimony of an expert witness also may be used against the nurse.

Following are five areas that potentially can increase liability for the nurse (Dernovsek et al., 2001)

- **Failure to ensure patient safety**
  Examples include inappropriate assessment and triage, not following guidelines as written, and lack of follow-up as needed.
- **Failure to communicate**
  The nurse always must listen to the patient and avoid jumping to conclusions or leading the caller. Convey information in a manner the caller can understand, clarify information, and verify that the information is understood. It is essential to document the interaction and any follow-up calls.
- **Failure to follow policies and procedures**
  The nurse must be familiar with and understand the policies and procedures. These should be updated on a regular basis to match current practice and standards.
- **Failure to act on professional judgment**
  Abandoning professional judgment just to follow a guideline or protocol is not appropriate. The nurse must be able to show that professional judgment was used in every call.

- **Failure to document**
  Careful, clear documentation is required that would allow the nurse to re-create the call if needed for medical or legal reasons.

The best way to protect yourself from legal risk is to carefully follow your facility's policies and procedures, which should be based on current standards of practice, including clinical practice guidelines, nurse practice acts, and any state laws relating to telephone triage. Even if your facility does not have a formal telephone triage program, you often will find yourself giving advice over the telephone. Patients will continue to call looking for advice and information. It is not practical to believe you can deny this service to your patients. Buppert (2002), attorney at law, recommended that clinicians not provide telephone care unless the patient has been seen by the practice and the patient's chart is at hand with a recorded medical history, baseline examination, and current contact information in the chart. It is key to realize that Buppert is not denying the nurse's duty to respond to the patient once the call is answered, rather that telephone advice should not be provided. It would not be reasonable to do so without any knowledge of the patient. The patient should be referred to a local ED or family physician, or an appointment at a clinic should be made. Buppert emphasized that the advice given should be documented with the patient's complaint and history. This should be completed before the end of the day. Finally, the patient should be given an appointment for follow-up. Buppert cautioned nurses that it is important to direct the patient immediately to call 911 for emergency situations, such as chest pain or dyspnea.

Strategies to Minimize Liability

There are ways in which legal risk can be reduced even before a nurse answers a call. These involve development of appropriate policies, procedures, and guidelines. There should be a clear statement of the purpose and goals of telephone triage. This should include the limits of services, as well as the goals the telephone triage nurse is expected to meet. The job description should accurately explain the role of the nurse in telephone triage, describe the scope of practice, and include minimum qualifications (a minimum of three years of RN experience in an applicable clinical area prior to telehealth nursing is the telephone triage industry standard) (Espensen, 2001). It should detail accountability for outcomes and should be reviewed annually to ensure it reflects current responsibilities and evolving standards of telephone nursing.

Policies and procedures should be developed and regularly reviewed to ensure they reflect current standards. It is important that policies and procedures should not be written with unattainable expectations, such as that all telephone calls will be answered within three rings or every patient is seen within 24 hours. Policies and procedures are guidelines that direct the nurse's practice.

To further reduce risk, policies should be developed to manage anticipated problem situations, and these should delineate the procedures to be used.

Depending on the setting, policies should be developed to cover the following issues (list is not all-inclusive).

- Communication with minors
- Noncompliant callers
- Angry or obscene callers
- Inability to contact patient or caller
- Anonymous callers
- Third-party callers—neighbors or others calling on behalf of the patient with or without the patient's permission
- Conversations with the caller instead of with the patient
- Calls from caregivers
- Refusal to provide medical history
- Language barriers, including how to manage the hearing-impaired patient
- Backup technology (computer and telephone lines)
- Access to emergency medical service
- Referrals to providers and services
- Confidentiality of the call and documentation
- Out-of-state calls
- Out-of-country calls
- Prioritizing calls by call type and severity
- Types of calls to accept (e.g., triage, prescription)
- Patients who call who are not your patients
- Multiple symptom calls and clinical guidelines to use
- Overriding guidelines
- Symptoms that do not fit any of your written protocols
- Providing over-the-counter medication dosages
- New prescriptions and refills
- Lab test ordering and disclosing results
- Elderly abuse/neglect
- Child abuse/neglect
- Ingestions and poisoning
- Suicide or psychiatric calls
- Chronic callers

In addition to policy and procedure development, other measures can be taken in developing telephone triage within your practice to minimize risk. The following section discusses some of these strategies.

Select, maintain, and rely on protocols or guidelines. Guidelines are not "cookbook" medicine but rather a guide to manage the telephone call in a manner that is safe and congruent with nursing and physician practice. AAACN (2001a) and the American Association of Office Nurses (AAON, n.d.) have established standards that outline the use of written guidelines. A court of law may find informal telephone triage unacceptable when the nurse provides information "off the top of his or her head." Guidelines should be developed and/or adopted from another source. The appropriate physician should approve and regularly review all guidelines and changes. The physician has the ultimate responsibility for the care of patients, and his or her input should be sought and valued. Remember, although the physician oversees the guidelines, these are developed for the professional nurse and are not to be used as diagnostic tools. These guidelines should include when a caller should be referred for immediate services, such as a call to 911 or instructions to the patient to proceed immediately to a local ED, or emergent services so a physician sees the patient the same day the call is received.

When a nurse applies a guideline, it is extremely important to document the guideline used as a source and to read the information during the call rather than relying on memory. This enhances the quality of the communication by improving adherence to the established guidelines. It also decreases liability because if the information were challenged in court, it would be easy to recreate the response and defend the action that was taken. Calls should be documented in a manner that makes it possible to recreate the call. Documentation should include but not be limited to protocols used, the patient's complaint in the patient's words, the information the nurse gleaned from the assessment interview, a detailed description of the information given to the patient, including when and how to seek care, the resources used, referrals made and reason for the referrals, confirmation that the patient demonstrated understanding of the information/instructions, and that the patient found the advice acceptable. Brief narrative notes may not be adequate; a standardized form may assist the nurse in establishing cues to complete documentation. Checking boxes for specific phrases can strengthen the documentation. The nurse should make notes throughout the call and complete the documentation record immediately following the conclusion of the call.

Managing telephone calls can consume hours of each working day, yet the call volume can fluctuate from hour to hour and day to day. The call volumes should be monitored to ensure that appropriate staff is available to respond in a timely fashion. The practice should define adequate staffing levels for peak and off-peak calling times. Symptom-based calls should never be left until the next day, as this could be considered abandonment of care.

The telephone triage nurse must be knowledgeable in the specialty and have additional resources necessary, such as reference materials, published standards of practice, facility policies, procedures, and guidelines. If the office is paperless and the medical record and/or guidelines are available in a computer, a backup plan should be developed to cover times when the computer is not available.

Risk may be reduced when the patient is satisfied with the telephone call; a satisfied patient is less likely to sue. The greatest complaint in surveys that looked at telephone triage was the length of time it took the caller to connect with the nurse (Moore, Saywell, Thakker, & Jones, 2002). Notifying callers immediately that they may have to wait to speak to a nurse enhances caller satisfaction and may reduce the risk of a lawsuit. If the triage nurse needs to return the call, it is best to provide the caller with an estimate of when his or her call will be returned. This estimated time should be accurate based on the limits of the staff in the practice, and the caller should find it acceptable. If the caller states it is an emergency, he or she should be instructed to hang up and call 911. Always inform the patient that you are a nurse and cannot diagnose or prescribe. If the patient is insistent on speaking to a physician, this should not be denied. Avoid empty promises such as "everything will be all right" because this will only worsen the situation in the event of a negative outcome.

A follow-up phone call may be necessary to check on patient status, compliance, or understanding of instructions. There should be clear policies written to identify who should receive follow-up phone calls. A nurse may be inclined to make follow-up phone calls on a favorite patient. This favoritism raises legal risk because it can be interpreted as providing a different level of service to certain patients.

Quality assurance programs should be implemented to monitor interactions with patients and improve performance. Skill validations may include the nurse's ability to complete a thorough assessment, triage a call, communicate, and document. If the quality assurance program includes taping of calls, the caller must be informed and permission granted before the taping begins.

PATIENT CONFIDENTIALITY

Patient confidentiality must be protected at all times. The patient has the same rights to protection of privacy and confidentiality over the telephone as he or she has when seen in the office. All policies and procedures employed in the office designed to meet privacy standards, including HIPAA requirements, need to extend to telephone services.

The HIPAA Privacy Rule (Department of Health and Human Services, 2003) has created national standards to protect individuals' medical records and other personal health information. It allows patients to have more control over their health information; it sets boundaries on the use and release of health records; it establishes appropriate safeguards that healthcare providers and others must follow to protect the privacy of health information; and it holds violators accountable with civil and criminal penalties. The HIPAA rule permits healthcare providers to communicate with patients regarding their health care. Many practices have written policies and procedures to address these HIPAA requirements.

These policies and procedures should outline with whom, if anyone, in addition to the patient, the nurse may discuss the patient's care. Some oncology practices are requiring the patient to sign a form designating, if desired, any other specific individual to which the patient's medical information may be provided. If the patient has not provided permission, no information would be shared with anyone but the patient.

Additional measures have been taken by some practices to ensure the identity of a caller. The patient and significant other, with permission to discuss the patient's care, are provided with a password. This helps to verify the caller's identity over the phone.

Follow-up calls from the nurse to check on the status of the patient, to monitor patient compliance, or to provide the patient with information raise new issues with caller identification (ID) systems and answering machines. The HIPAA rule does not prohibit leaving messages for the patients on their answering machines or with family members. However, it does require that reasonable safeguards are taken to guard the individual's privacy, and the information left should be limited. For example, leave only the name and number of the physician or nurse calling and limited information necessary to confirm an appointment or a return call.

Policies should be written to address appropriate use of caller ID displays, answering machines, voice mail, e-mail, and fax. In some clinics, patients are asked to sign authorization for the healthcare providers to leave information on a work or home answering machine, fax, or e-mail correspondence.

It is important that others do not overhear the conversation the nurse has with the patient. An appropriate workspace or office should be available for the telephone triage nurse. This is to ensure that patients or others do not overhear confidential information. The HIPAA rule does not require soundproof walls or structural changes to facilities; however, it requires that appropriate administrative, technical, and physical safeguards be taken to protect the privacy of the patient's health information.

The record of the telephone call and interaction is confidential whether it is on paper or computerized and should be protected in the same manner as the medical record. It is ideal to place all documentation on the call in the patient's medical record immediately and not to leave it lying about for others to see.

COMMUNICATING WITH SPECIAL POPULATIONS

Some populations have inherent barriers that nurses must overcome to communicate effectively. It is the nurse's responsibility to overcome barriers by communicating in a manner that the patient can understand regardless of age, mental disability, language barriers, domestic disturbances, or lack of access to an adult.

Minors

Minor callers pose a special challenge because they have special needs related to communication and consent. Legal definitions of minors vary from state to state. Nurses should verify policies and practices with their state's laws. Minors may call for several reasons. They could call with their own symptoms, on behalf of a peer or family member, or as a spokesperson for a family member who does not speak English. Policies should be developed to define what types of calls are accepted from minors and the information that can be provided.

Language Barriers

Nurses should be prepared to manage calls from patients with a language barrier, including those who do not speak English, have limited English, or are hearing impaired. If your practice does not have access to a translator for the non-English-speaking or a Telecommunications Device for the Deaf (TDD), your office should inform the patients with this special need on their first visit. Attempting to provide telephone services to these patients may be inappropriate without the proper support.

To reduce legal risks of misinterpretation, a translator service that understands medical terms should be used. When a family member or employee from down the hall is used to interpret, the information shared may need to be restricted, and there is no assurance that the information was portrayed accurately. When an informed consent is required, a translator service should be used to avoid legal risk. This holds true not only in translation of a foreign language but also for a sign translator if the patient is hearing impaired. If the office is equipped with a TDD, the staff should be instructed on and competent in its use.

Cultural and Socioeconomic Differences

Social taboos may prevent discussion of certain health problems or bar direct communication with certain family members. Some cultures will restrict discussion directly with the patient and require that the husband speak for the wife. Strategies need to be developed to address these and other challenges, including ones to help the patient who has poor vocabulary skills; cultural taboos that may make it difficult to talk about bodily functions; and how to manage patients with limited access to telephones, transportation, and healthcare support.

Calls to Be Handled With Caution

A patient's friend or family member calls seeking advice. Adhere to the policies related to which callers you provide telephone advice. Remember, a friendly neighbor today may not be so friendly in court if given the wrong information. Advise the family member or friend to contact their family healthcare provider or call 911 if it is an emergency.

Parents of ill children often are anxious over even the smallest of maladies and sometimes are unconcerned by potentially dangerous conditions. These attitudes can lead to misinformation. Parents of a child with cancer are more likely to suffer these feelings. They may call over every ache and pain or ignore a potentially life-threatening event, such as a temperature elevation. It is important to provide straightforward instructions without being judgmental.

The elderly are more susceptible to comorbidities complicating their cancer care. A thorough medical history that is verified with the patient to ensure it is up to date is key to managing this call. Often the elderly are reluctant to share information or seek help. They do not want to "bother" the physician or nurse, or they may feel their illness or complaint is a threat to their continued independence. When an elderly patient calls, it is imperative that the nurse provides time and attention to the caller, communicating an unhurried attitude to encourage the patient to share important information. Also, as many elderly patients experience some hearing loss, it is key that the nurse ensures that he or she can be heard and understood. Asking open-ended questions and being alert for the appropriateness of the answer can aid this.

The triage nurse may find himself or herself lacking patience with the frequent, chronic, or repeat caller. You must be aware of this inclination because a patient who calls often may call one day with a serious malady, and it may be missed. Listen to each call seriously prior to making any conclusions. If a patient calls repeatedly in one day with the same complaint, it is a good practice to bring that patient in to see the physician. If the symptom is not so acute to warrant a same-day appointment, certainly the anxiety it is causing the patient is.

If the assessment portion of the triage call is too short or too long, a red flag should go up in the nurse's mind. If the assessment portion of the call goes on for more than 10 minutes, this should be a warning that this patient should be seen. If the assessment is less than three minutes, the nurse and caller have not shared enough information to adequately assess the situation and triage appropriately (Dernovsek et al., 2001).

CLINICAL COMPETENCY

In general, the competencies required to provide safe and effective telephone triage mirror the competencies required of the professional nurse. The telephone triage nurse should have competencies related to the technologies being used and determine if these technologies are appropriate for the patient. It may not be appropriate to provide a follow-up telephone assessment of a patient who is hearing impaired if a TDD is not available or to e-mail patient instructions if the patient does not have ready access to and competency with a computer and the Internet. The hearing-impaired patient will need an appointment to be seen in the office, or the patient instructions will need to be faxed or mailed rather than e-mailed. In addition to technical knowledge, the professional nurse must have refined communication skills, possess an appropriate level of clinical expertise, and have good assessment skills.

Formal education of the nurse, including orientation and continuing education, will strengthen his or her telephone triage skills. Orientation should include aspects of assessing a patient without face-to-face contact, triaging using the clinical guidelines, communication skills, and documentation requirements and pitfalls. The industry average orientation period for a telephone triage nurse is two to four weeks (Espensen, 2001). The orientation process and continuing education should be documented in the nurse's personnel record. This is a requirement for accrediting bodies such as JCAHO.

The College of Registered Nurses of Nova Scotia (2000) has identified requisite competencies for RNs. Key competencies include

1. Establishing therapeutic nurse-patient relationships using the nursing process
2. Considering patients' cultural (including language), spiritual, and psychosocial needs and preferences
3. Collaborating with other members of healthcare teams, as appropriate and required, to ensure quality care and effective service
4. Providing nursing services consistent with the Standards for Nursing Practice, Code of Ethics, and Nurse Practice Act
5. Protecting the confidentiality and security of patient information and ensuring the privacy of interactions by developing and/or implementing appropriate policies
6. Delivering competent nursing services by assessing their own competence, identifying areas for learning, and addressing knowledge gaps relative to the technologies and nursing services provided
7. Documenting nurse:patient interactions
8. Supporting evidence-based practice by evaluating the effectiveness of services and modifying and improving practices accordingly.

Continued competency for the telephone triage nurse includes seeking avenues to ensure that their clinical and technical competencies are current. In this ever-growing subspecialty of nursing care, the professional nurse needs to pay particular attention to the changing legal environment of telephone nursing. This includes, but is not limited to, state board practice decisions and licensure issues.

As an emerging field, telenursing may require additional education to support competent practice; however, few formal educational programs are available. AAACN has published *Telehealth Nursing Practice Administration and Practice Standards* (2001a) and offers a course and manual on telehealth nursing practice (2001b). This course is designed to meet the needs of nurses practicing telephone nursing in telephone triage centers. However, the information is general, and much of it can be applied to the oncology nurse. More information regarding the standards, the course, and the manual is available on the AAACN Web site (www.aaacn.org). In addition, the National Certification Corporation (2001) now offers a Telephone Nursing Practice Certification. More information about the certification can be found on their Web site (www.nccnet.org).

CONCLUSION

In the 1800s, two individuals changed the world of nursing care when they introduced their innovations. Florence Nightingale brought reform to the nursing profession, bringing to it dignity and science while across the sea; Alexander Graham Bell made his first call on his new invention—the telephone. The author does not believe Bell or Nightingale could foresee that the telephone would someday become a tool for nurses, a tool that permits increased access to patients and allows the nurse to apply the nursing process from a distance.

Triage, a process first employed at the battlefield to allocate limited resources, is now a process employed in EDs and clinics everywhere. Oncology nurses use telephone triage not only to evaluate the critical nature of a patient's complaint and provide appropriate disposition advice but also to listen to and assess patient complaints and provide emotional support and homecare education.

Telephone nursing has created new challenges in oncology nursing. Nurses have been educated in clinical settings, allowing full use of their five senses, whereas the telephone limits sensory input. Communication challenges include how to elicit the most information in a clear and concise manner without leading the caller. Process challenges exist within the busy clinic setting. The volume and nature of telephone calls are unpredictable. It is important to provide time and attention to the caller, but how is that best balanced with the time and attention needed for the patients physically present? Models of telephone triage vary significantly depending on the size of the clinic and staffing patterns. Legal challenges include those related to state licensure issues. When the call is initiated beyond state borders, in which state should the nurse hold licensure? A number of processes and tips can help in limiting legal liabilities, including the appropriate use of telephone triage policies, guidelines or protocols, and documentation.

This text has provided an overview of telephone triage or telephone nursing as it exists today in oncology clinics across this nation. It has sought to address communication tips and suggestions for triage processes. The authors discussed legal concerns and dynamic issues that will require the nurses' ongoing vigilance of state and national regulations. Additionally, suggestions on ways to limit liability have been addressed. The next section contains sample telephone protocols focusing on common complaints of patients with cancer. These protocols result from a review of the current nursing literature and contributions of protocols used by nurses from across the United States. It is imperative that all telephone protocols used in each unique clinic setting be reviewed and approved by the supervising physician in the practice.

Oncology nursing is a dynamic process focused on providing patient care to patients and families experiencing a cancer diagnosis. The authors hope that this text will assist our nursing colleagues in their quest to provide quality care in today's fast-moving, technologically advanced world.

REFERENCES

American Academy of Ambulatory Care Nursing. (2001a). *Telehealth nursing practice administration and practice standards.* Pitman, NJ: Jannetti.

American Academy of Ambulatory Care Nursing. (2001b). *Telehealth nursing practice core course manual.* Pitman, NJ: Jannetti.

American Association of Office Nurses. (n.d.). *Office nursing practice standards for quality care of patients.* Retrieved January 5, 2004, from http://www.aaon.org/pract.html

American College of Emergency Physicians. (2000). *ACEP position statement: Providing telephone advice from the emergency department.* Retrieved June 22, 2003, from http://www.acep.org/1,658,0.html

American Nurses Association. (1996). *Telehealth issues for nursing.* ANA policy series. Retrieved January 12, 2004, from http://nursingworld.org/readingroom.tele2.htm

Arkansas State Board of Nursing. (2000, October/November). *Telenursing position statement adopted.* Retrieved July 5, 2003, from http://www.state.ar.us/nurse

Buppert, C. (2002, August 19). *Avoiding the risks of diagnosing and treating by phone. The Gold Sheet.* Retrieved April 27, 2003, from http://www.medscape.com/viewarticle/439162

California State Board of Nursing. (2001, September). *RN tele-nursing and telephone triage.* Retrieved July 5, 2003, from http://www.dca.ca.gov/tmas

College of Registered Nurses of Nova Scotia. (2000, November). *Guidelines for telenursing practice.* Retrieved July 5, 2003, from http://www.crnns.ca/documents/telenursing.pdf

Department of Health and Human Services. (2003, April). *Protecting the privacy of patients' health information.* Retrieved January 5, 2004, from http://www.hhs.gov/news/facts/privacy.html

Dernovsek, D., Espensen, M., & Massengale, A. (2001). *Session 107: Legal aspects of telehealth nursing: Telehealth nursing practice core course manual.* (2001). Pitman, NJ: Jannetti.

Emergency Nurses Association. (2001). *ENA position statement: Telephone advice.* Retrieved June 22, 2003, from http://www.ena.org/about/position/telephoneadvice.asp

Espensen, M. (2001). *Telehealth nursing practice. AAACN core curriculum for ambulatory care nursing.* St. Louis, MO: Harcourt Health Services.

Hutcherson, C., & Williamson, S. (1999, May 31). Nursing regulation for the new millennium: The mutual recognition model. *Online Journal of Issues in Nursing.* Retrieved June 19, 2003, from http://www.nursingworld.org/ojin/topic9/topic9_2htm

Kabala, E.J. (1998, September). Legalities of a telephone nurse triage system. *Physician's News Digest.* Retrieved July 5, 2003, from http://www.physiciansnews.com/law/998Kabala.html

Marker-Smith, C. (1988). *Setting standards for professional nursing: The Marker Model.* St. Louis, MO: Mosby.

Merriam-Webster's Medical Dictionary. (2003). Retrieved January 5, 2004, from http://www.intelihealth.com

Moore, J.D., Saywell, R.M., Thakker, N., & Jones, T.A. (2002). An analysis of patient compliance with nurse recommendations from after hours call centers. *American Journal of Managed Care, 8,* 343–351.

National Certification Corporation. (2001). *Facts about the NCC 2001 telephone nursing practice certification examination.* Retrieved July 5, 2003, from http://www.ehealthnurse.com/ncc_tn.html

National Council of State Boards of Nursing. (1997, August). *Position paper on telenursing: A challenge to regulation.* Retrieved June 19, 2003, from http://www.ncsbn.org/public/news/res/telenursing

National Council of State Boards of Nursing. (1998, November 6). *Revised approved interstate compact language.* Retrieved July 5, 2003, from http://www.ncsbn.org/files/msrtf/compact9811.pdf

National Council of State Boards of Nursing. (2003, April). *Nurse licensure compact.* Retrieved August 17, 2003, from http://www.ncsbn.org/public/nurselicensurecompact/mutual_recognition_state.htm

Nevada State Board of Nursing. (2002, October). *Committee News.* Retrieved July 6, 2003, from http://www.state.nv.us/boards/nsbn/Newsletters/October%202002.pdf

Telephone Triage Guidelines

Alopecia

PROBLEM

Loss of hair

ASSESSMENT CRITERIA

1. What is the cancer diagnosis and treatment?
   a. Hair loss (alopecia) is the most obvious consequence of cancer treatment and also is one of the most distressing of all the potential treatment side effects. It is the hallmark sign that someone has cancer. It can arouse enough anxiety to cause some patients to refuse treatment.
   b. Many cancer treatments work by targeting rapidly growing cancer cells. This action is responsible for most cancer treatment side effects. Hair follicles are among the many fast-growing healthy cells in the body.
   c. Certain chemotherapy drugs and radiation therapy will cause partial or total hair loss. There are two phases of hair growth, the active growing phase and the resting or dormant phase. Cancer therapy affects hair in the active phase only. The surface of the head has 85% of the 100,000 total hair follicles in the active growing phase, which is why hair on the head falls out first. Hair on the face, underarms, pubic area, and legs have more follicles in the resting phase, so it may take longer to notice hair loss in these areas (Larkin, 2002).
2. What medication(s) is the patient taking? Obtain drug history.
   Chronic use of other drugs, such as steroids, also causes thinning of hair.

HOMECARE INSTRUCTIONS

When will hair loss occur?

Chemotherapy

Hair loss depends on the type of chemotherapy used and the growth rate and condition of the patient's hair. The drug, dose, and timing of the treatments will affect the rate of hair loss. People with less hair in the active growing phase tend to have less hair loss. Permanents, hair straightening agents, and hair dyes weaken hair, making hair loss more likely. Hair loss usually occurs two to three weeks after the first dose of chemotherapy. Permanent hair loss is extremely rare. Hair begins to grow back four to six weeks after the last dose of chemotherapy (DeVita, Hellman, & Rosenberg, 2001). Patients usually report burning one to two days before hair begins to fall out. Hair may come out in clumps.

Radiation Therapy

Hair follicles are affected by radiation therapy, which also targets rapidly dividing cells. Radiation therapy is directed locally, so hair is lost only in the areas directly in its path (where it enters and exits) and not on shielded locations. The extent of hair loss depends upon the dose of radiation. Hair loss begins two to three weeks after radiation treatments begin. Hair usually grows back three to six months after standard dose radiation (5,000 to 6,000 cGy) is complete. High-dose radiation (6,000 cGy or more) may cause permanent hair loss (Robbins & Gosselin, 2002). Patients should be cautioned that the new hair may have a different color and texture, also true of chemotherapy.

Tips During Hair Loss (Intermountain Health Care, 2003; National Institutes of Health, 1999)

- Visit a hair stylist prior to treatment. Hair loss often is better managed by cutting the hair short prior to treatment.
- Shop for a wig in advance of hair loss. It is best to shop for a wig before hair is lost in order to match hair color, style, and texture. It is important to have some sort of head covering to protect the skin from sun and wind.
- Use a sunscreen on exposed scalp or cover completely to protect skin from the sun's harmful rays.
- Sleep on a soft, satiny pillowcase to minimize friction.
- Keep hair clean by shampooing with a gentle, pH-balanced shampoo. Avoid vigorous toweling and blow-drying any remaining hair.
- Use a soft-bristle brush or a wide-toothed comb.
- Avoid hair treatments such as bleaching, permanents, hair dye, and hair spray that can cause dry or brittle hair.
- Try not to braid hair or put in a ponytail.
- Wear a turban at night to keep hair from collecting on pillows.

Report the Following Problems

- If your scalp becomes irritated
- If you have experienced prolonged sun exposure
- If your skin is red, itchy, and swollen

REFERENCES

DeVita, V., Hellman, S., & Rosenberg, S. (2001). *Cancer: Principles and practice of oncology* (6th ed.). Philadelphia: Lippincott Williams & Wilkins.

Intermountain Health Care. (2003). *Symptom management: Hair loss.* Retrieved June 30, 2003, from http://ihc.cancersource.com

Larkin, L. (2002). *Side effect management series: Hair loss.* Retrieved February 12, 2004, from http://www.oncology.com

National Institutes of Health. (1999). *Chemotherapy and you. A guide to self-help during cancer treatment.* Retrieved February 12, 2004, from http://www.nci.nih.gov/cancerinfo/chemotherapy-and-you

Robbins, M., & Gosselin, T.K. (2002). Symptom management in radiation oncology. Acute and long-term side effects. *American Journal of Nursing, 102*(Suppl. 4), 32–36.

Linda Bracks-Madison, RN, BSN

Clinical Nurse, Outpatient

University of Texas M.D. Anderson Cancer Center

Houston, TX

Alterations in Sexuality

PROBLEM

Inability to enjoy sexual activity (Bruner & Berk, 2004)

ASSESSMENT CRITERIA

Start with less sensitive questions and move toward more sensitive ones. Provide patient with a confidentiality statement concerning conversation. Advise patient that he or she may choose not to answer sensitive questions.

1. What is the history of cancer and subsequent cancer treatment?
2. What are the coexisting variables?
    a. Gender
    b. Age
    c. Educational background
    d. Socioeconomic status
    e. Cultural or ethnic background
    f. Concurrent medical or psychiatric disorders
    g. Current prescription and over-the-counter medication use
3. How has the diagnosis or cancer treatment changed your sexual function and your feelings about your body?
4. Has the role with your partner changed since you were diagnosed with or treated for cancer? If yes, how has the role changed?
5. Using the ALARM Model for Assessment of Sexual Functioning, assess for Activity, Libido/Desire, Arousal and Orgasm, Resolution, and Medical history (Andersen, 1990).
    a. Activity: How frequent are the current sexual activities? Are other forms of physical affection, such as hugging or kissing, being communicated?
    b. Libido/desire: How has the desire and interest for sexual activity changed, either in initiating or responding to your partner?
    c. Arousal and orgasm: When sexually excited, does the penis become erect or vagina lubricated, followed by ejaculation or vaginal contractions?
    d. Resolution: Following sexual activity, is there a release of sexual tension and a satisfaction with sexual life?
    e. Medical history: Are there any acute or chronic disorders that may interfere with sexual activity, such as diabetes, hypertension, substance abuse, or psychiatric disorders?

HOMECARE INSTRUCTIONS

Action and approach are dependent on patient response to assessment questions. A common method used to manage alterations in sexual health is the PLISSIT model (Annon, 1974). The model uses a four-step approach to deal with sexual concerns: permission, limited information, specific suggestions, and intensive therapy. The majority of sexual problems related to cancer can be managed without referral for intensive therapy.

Permission

Many patients are uncomfortable discussing sexual concerns. Therefore, it is up to the healthcare provider to initiate the conversation and provide permission to discuss concerns.

Limited Information

Provide information about how cancer therapy will affect sexual functioning.

Specific Suggestions

Interventions can be suggested for the specific problems identified through the assessment process. The methods for dealing with altered sexual health include suggesting new ways of sexual expression, new sexual positions, and new communication patterns. The American Cancer Society offers various resources to facilitate coping with sexual changes related to cancer.

Report the Following Problems

Notify physician if no improvement has occurred. A referral for more intensive therapy may be indicated. Providers for more intensive therapy may include a surgeon, gynecologist, urologist, social worker, psychologist, psychiatrist, or sex therapist.

REFERENCES

Andersen, B. (1990). How cancer affects sexual functioning. *Oncology, 4,* 81–88.
Annon, J. (1974). *The behavioral treatment of sexual problems.* Honolulu, HI: Kapiolani Health Services
Bruner, D.W., & Berk, L. (2004). Altered body image and sexual health. In C.H. Yarbro, M.H. Frogge, & M. Goodman (Eds.), *Cancer symptom management* (3rd ed., pp. 596–635). Sudbury, MA: Jones and Bartlett.

Joyce Marrs, RN, BSN, OCN®
Staff Nurse
Medical Oncology Hematology Associates, Inc.
Dayton, OH

Anorexia

PROBLEM

An aversion to food, associated with significant weight loss. When the daily physiologic demands exceed the person's dietary consumption, the body's reserves are used to meet energy and protein needs (Brown, 2002).

ASSESSMENT CRITERIA

1. What is the cancer diagnosis and treatment? Is the person in advanced stages of the disease (Cope, 2002)?
2. What medication(s) is the patient taking? Obtain drug history.
3. Ask patient to describe symptoms in detail (total amount of weight loss over what period of time).
4. Obtain history, including
   a. Precipitating factors: weight patterns, gain and loss cycles, nutritional intake patterns, and whether weighed on a single scale or on several different scales
   b. Onset and duration
   c. Relieving factors
   d. Any associated symptoms such as nausea and vomiting, weakness, fatigue, amenorrhea, polyuria, or cold intolerance.
5. Past medical history (e.g., eating disorders)
6. Changes in activities of daily living

Signs and Symptoms	Action
• Lack of nutritional intake for several days • Orthostatic hypotension (dizziness when standing)	Seek urgent care within two to four hours.
• Weight loss > 5% of baseline in one month • Minimal nutritional intake for several days • Continual loss of weight, despite adherence to instructions and ingestion of supplements and prescribed appetite stimulants	Obtain appointment to see medical professional within a few days.

(Continued on next page)

(Continued)

Signs and Symptoms	Action
• Weight loss > 10% of baseline in six months (Whitman, 2000)	Yes—Obtain appointment to see medical professional within a week. No—Continue nutritional program, supplements, appetite stimulants, and other homecare instructions.
Cross references: Depressed Mood, Dysphagia, Nausea and Vomiting, Xerostomia	

HOMECARE INSTRUCTIONS

- Avoid strong food odors or foods that are not appetizing.
- Try cold foods, such as smoothies, sandwiches, and yogurt.
- Eat several small meals per day.
- Fortify milk by adding powdered milk.
- Add protein supplements or powdered milk to casseroles, smoothies, etc.
- Sip on nutritious drinks, such as fruit juices, when thirsty.
- Eat the most when you feel the hungriest, regardless of the time of day.
- Eat nutritious high-protein foods, such as fish, lean meat, eggs, and nuts.
- Add supplements such as Ensure® (Abbott Laboratories, Abbott Park, IL)/ProSure® (Abbott Laboratories), two cans per day (Guenter, Ferguson, Thrush, & Voss, 2002).
- Consult dietitian or homecare instruction sheet for recipes and suggestions.
- Take an appetite stimulant, such as Marinol® (Solvay Pharmaceuticals, Marietta, GA) or Megace® (Bristol-Myers Squibb, Princeton, NJ), if prescribed.
- Take antiemetics, if prescribed, for nausea.
- Remain as active as possible, utilizing mild exercise, such as walking or swimming.
- Practice relaxation exercises 30 minutes before meals to decrease stress.

Report the Following Problems

- Continued lack of appetite with little or no food ingestion
- Continued weight loss
- Uncontrolled nausea that interferes with the ability to eat

Seek Emergency Care Immediately if the Following Occurs

- Fainting when changing from a sitting to a standing position

REFERENCES

Brown, J.K. (2002). A systematic review of the evidence on symptom management of cancer-related anorexia and cachexia. *Oncology Nursing Forum, 29,* 517–532.

Cope, D.G. (2002). Management of anorexia, cachexia, and weight loss in patients with advanced cancer. *Clinical Journal of Oncology Nursing, 6,* 241–242.

Guenter, P., Ferguson, M., Thrush, K., & Voss, A.C. (2002). Understanding tumor-induced weight loss. *Medsurg Nursing, 11,* 215–227.

Whitman, M.M. (2000). The starving patient: Supportive care for people with cancer. *Clinical Journal of Oncology Nursing, 14,* 121–125.

Pat Reymann, RN, MSN, AOCN®
Oncology Consultant
Birmingham, AL

Anxiety

PROBLEM

Apprehension of danger accompanied by restlessness, tension, tachycardia, and dyspnea unattached to a clearly identifiable stimulus.

ASSESSMENT CRITERIA

Signs and Symptoms	Action

• Determine if the patient is experiencing anxiety.
  - Physical symptoms
    ♦ Shortness of breath, palpitations, dry mouth, flushing of the face, dizziness, tingling, trembling, sleep disturbance, headache, and muscular tension
	Establish trust by reassuring the patient that you are there to help. Conduct the interview in a calm and nonjudgmental manner. Allow self-expression without patient feeling rushed, and assist with thought processes if the patient is unable to recall events in a logical manner.

- Psychological symptoms ♦ Feeling of apprehension, comorbid depression, excessive worry, inability to relax, fear of losing control, fear of dying, inability to think clearly, cognitive over-arousal, irritability, avoidance, or agoraphobia	Ask about the patient's perception of general health, pain, disability level, or immediate danger. Have these perceptions recently changed? Is the anxiety related to a recent event or a general sense of foreboding?
• Determine if the patient can receive intervention safely via telephone for the interim.	Call 911 if patient or others are in immediate danger. Otherwise, have the patient take prescribed anxiolytics. Ask what coping mechanisms have helped in the past, and suggest methods such as biofeedback, relaxation techniques, soft music, and/or deep breathing. If applicable, initiate a supportive counsel consult or a clinic visit and/or notify MD.

(Continued on next page)

(Continued)

Signs and Symptoms	Action
• Determine sources of support: - Is a family member present or readily accessible? - Is the patient established with a counselor?	Activate the support system by talking with a family member, if one is with the patient, or call an identified support person or counselor. If needed, initiate a supportive counsel consult or a clinic visit and/or notify MD.
• Determine medicine/substance-related factors: - Has the patient recently started new medications that can cause restlessness or anxiety? - Has the patient recently changed intake of alcohol, caffeine, nicotine, or illicit drugs? - Does the patient use anxiogenic, thyroid, or psychostimulant medications or herbal remedies such as ma-huang?	Assess whether the drug can produce paradoxical or sympathetic responses. If so, explain the link between anxiety and physiologic response to medications. Some examples are benzodiazepines (lorazepam, alprazolam, clonazepam, diazepam, temazepam, and flurazepam), antihistamines (hydroxyzine and diphenhydramine), phenothiazines (promethazine and prochlorperazine), dopaminergic antagonists (metoclopramide and haloperidol), steroids, and psychostimulants such as methylphenidate. If the medication can safely be discontinued, instruct the patient to stop the medication and call the primary physician or physician on call.
• Determine preexisting conditions that can elicit anxiety. - Does the patient's diagnosis increase risk for neurocognitive changes, such as cardiac history, pulmonary problems (hypoxia or dyspnea), comorbid depression, diabetes/hypoglycemia, intracranial metastases, uncontrolled pain, history of substance abuse or history of panic/anxiety attacks?	Assess if symptoms can be alleviated safely with telephone intervention. If unable to intervene successfully over the phone, refer the patient to appropriate medical intervention (e.g., page MD, go to ED, call 911 or ambulance service).
- Is the patient experiencing new stressors, such as social issues, insomnia, new medical diagnoses, disease progression, or grief/loss issues?	Allow the patient time for self-expression and provide supportive counseling. Assist with problem solving and provide numbers for counseling services. Communication should be empathetic and nonhurried.

(Continued on next page)

(Continued)

Signs and Symptoms	Action
- Does the patient have a history of major depression, post-traumatic stress disorder, schizophrenia, or generalized panic/anxiety attacks?	Notify MD and set up a clinic visit. Communicate appointment time to patient as soon as possible. Always make a follow-up phone call and arrange a clinic visit if the patient has responded to the telephone assistance. If unable to diminish anxiety, notify the physician, and arrange a clinic visit within the next 24 hours. If necessary, have the patient go to the nearest emergency room.

Note. Based on information from Bush, 1998; Elsayem & Bruera, 2002; Feldman & Christensen, 2003; Fisch & Bruera, 2003; Roesch et al., 2002; Sivesind & Baile, 2001.

HOMECARE INSTRUCTIONS

- Continue any current medications, especially medications prescribed for anxiety.
- Seek available support systems.
- Find methods to deal with increased anxiety (e.g., music/art therapy, exercise).
- Identify what may trigger feelings of anxiety.
- Learn relaxation breathing.

Report the Following Problems in 24 Hours

- Continued symptoms of anxiety despite use of medications and relaxation techniques
- Feelings of overwhelming sadness

Seek Emergency Care Immediately if Either of the Following Occurs

- Severe physical symptom uncontrolled with standard medication
- Feelings of loss of control with thoughts of suicide

REFERENCES

Bush, N.J. (1998). Anxiety and the cancer experience. In R.M. Carroll-Johnson, L.M. Gorman, & N.J. Bush (Eds.), *Psychosocial nursing care along the cancer continuum.* Pittsburgh, PA: Oncology Nursing Society.

Elsayem, A., & Bruera, E. (2002). *M.D. Anderson symptom control and palliative care handbook* (2nd ed.). Houston, TX: University of Texas-Houston Health Science Center.

Feldman, M., & Christensen, J. (2003). *Behavioral medicine in primary care: A practical guide*. New York: McGraw-Hill.

Fisch, M., & Bruera, E. (2003). *Handbook of advanced cancer care*. New York: Cambridge University Press.

Roesch, S., Weiner, B., & Vaughn, A. (2002). Cognitive approaches to stress and coping. *Current Opinion in Psychiatry, 15,* 627–632.

Sivesind, D., & Baile, W. (2001). The psychologic distress in patients with cancer. *Nursing Clinics of North America, 36,* 809–825.

Julie Snider, RN, BSN, OCN®
Clinical Coordinator
Department of Palliative Care and Rehabilitation Medicine
University of Texas M.D. Anderson Cancer Center
Houston, TX

Mary Murphy, RN, MS, AOCN®, CHPN
Director of Clinical Systems/Hospice Clinical Nurse Specialist
Hospice of Dayton
Dayton, OH

Ascites

PROBLEM

Accumulation of fluid within the peritoneal cavity

ASSESSMENT CRITERIA

(Marincola & Schwartzengruber, 2001; Winkelman, 2004)

1. What is the cancer diagnosis and treatment?
   Malignant ascites occurs commonly with intra-abdominal malignancies such as ovarian, colon, lymphoma, mesothelioma, stomach, liver, fallopian tube, and pancreatic. May also occur as a result of metastatic disease to the liver.
2. What medication(s) is the patient taking? Obtain drug history.
3. Ask patient to describe symptoms in detail.
   a. Abdominal or low back pain
   b. Abdominal fullness, pressure, or distension
   c. Urinary frequency or urgency
   d. Shortness of breath
   e. Decreased appetite or early satiety
   f. Weight gain
   g. Nausea
   h. Lower extremity edema
4. Obtain history, including
   a. Precipitating factors
   b. Onset and duration
   c. Relieving factors
   d. Any associated symptoms.
5. Past medical history (e.g., liver disease)
6. Changes in activities of daily living

Signs and Symptoms	Action
• Severe shortness of breath • Acute abdominal pain • Temperature of > 100.4°F with neutropenia • Unresponsiveness	Seek emergency care. Call ambulance immediately.

(Continued on next page)

ASCITES

(Continued)

Signs and Symptoms	Action
• Difficulty breathing • Abdominal discomfort • Weight gain > five pounds in past two days • Uncontrolled nausea and vomiting for more than 24 hours • Changes in mental status (increased somnolence) • Inability to perform activities of daily living (e.g., dressing, feeding, grooming, bathing, toileting)	Seek urgent care within two hours.
• Swelling of ankles • Inability to eat or drink fluids for 24 hours • Weight gain > five pounds in past week • Decrease in ability to perform activities of daily living (e.g., dressing, feeding, grooming, bathing, toileting) • Inability to sleep or rest due to shortness of breath or abdominal discomfort • Lack of bowel movement > three days beyond usual bowel elimination pattern	Seek care within 24 hours.
• Increased tightness of clothing in the abdominal area • Abdominal fullness, bloating, heaviness, or tightness • Indigestion • Increased frequency of voiding • Nausea or vomiting	Follow homecare instructions. Notify MD if no improvement.

Note. Based on information from Marincola & Schwartzengruber, 2001; Winkelman, 2004.

HOMECARE INSTRUCTIONS

(Marincola & Schwartzengruber, 2001; Winkelman, 2004)

Diet

- Eat six small, high-protein, high-caloric meals per day.
- Sit up for 30 minutes after each meal.
- Maintain fluid intake (3,000 cc per day).

Comfort

- Avoid wearing clothing that restricts the abdomen.
- Elevate head with pillows to ease work of breathing.

- Elevate lower extremities to reduce edema.
- Position for comfort.
- Use pressure reduction devices: mattress or heel protectors.

Activities of Daily Living

- Use assistive devices for picking up objects or ambulation.
- Use energy conservation techniques.
- Seek assistance from support network as needed.

Monitor for Critical Changes

- Weigh every other day.
- Take temperature once a day.
- Monitor urine output for changes in color (darker) or volume (decreased).
- Monitor for changes in skin over the abdomen and buttocks (increased redness, breakdown).

Report the Following Problems

- Lack of improvement in or presence of new signs and symptoms
- Acute changes in severity of signs and symptoms
- Decrease in ability to perform activities of daily living

Seek Emergency Care Immediately if Any of the Following Occurs

- Severe shortness of breath
- Acute abdominal pain
- Temperature of > 100.4°F
- Unresponsiveness

REFERENCES

Marincola, F.M., & Schwartzengruber, D.J. (2001). Malignant ascites. In V.T. DeVita, S. Hellman, & S.A. Rosenberg (Eds.), *Cancer: Principles and practice of oncology* (6th ed., pp. 2745–2752). Philadelphia: Lippincott Williams & Wilkins.

Winkelman, L.A. (2004). Malignant ascites. In C.H. Yarbro, M.H. Frogge, & M. Goodman (Eds.), *Cancer symptom management* (3rd ed., pp. 401–419). Sudbury, MA: Jones and Bartlett.

Jane Clark, PhD, RN, AOCN®, APRN-BC
Oncology Nursing Consultant
Decatur, GA

Bleeding

PROBLEM

Bleeding can occur secondary to injury or disease, including problems with coagulation resulting from use of anticoagulants or thrombocytopenia. It can be a life-threatening event if massive blood loss is allowed to occur.

ASSESSMENT CRITERIA

1. What is the cancer diagnosis and treatment?
   Bleeding can be caused by the tumor invading surrounding structures or blood vessels; the cancer may cause disseminated intravascular coagulation. Bleeding can be secondary to thrombocytopenia. Thrombocytopenia or a decreased number of platelets can result from the cancer or from disorders associated with splenomegaly, including non-Hodgkin's lymphoma, chronic lymphocytic leukemia, chronic liver disease, infection, or bone marrow injury secondary to the cancer, chemotherapy, and radiation therapy.
2. What medication(s) is the patient taking? Obtain drug history.
3. Obtain history of any active bleeding, including
   a. Precipitating factors—injury related or spontaneous
   b. Onset and duration—when did bleeding start, and how long has it persisted?
   c. Estimated amount of blood loss—describe how many feminine pads per hour if vaginal bleeding, how many bandages used.
   d. Relieving factors—is bleeding stopped or slowed with direct pressure or other homecare measures?
   e. Any associated symptoms, such as lightheadedness, pale skin color, cool or moist skin, thirst, or rapid pulse.
4. Ask patient to describe symptoms in detail.
   a. If active bleeding, is it slow and steady or spurting?
   b. If active bleeding from a wound, describe the wound.
   c. Petechiae—usually seen when platelet count drops below 20,000/mm^3 in dependent regions and over bony prominences (Lynch, 2000).
   d. Bruising
   e. Hemorrhagic vesicles inside the mouth or other mucous membranes
   f. Hematuria
   g. Gastrointestinal bleeding—melena, hematemesis

5. Past medical history (in addition to cancer history and cancer therapy)
   a. Use of anticoagulants
   b. Bleeding disorder
   c. New drugs used or exposure to toxic chemicals
6. Changes in activities of daily living

Signs and Symptoms	Action

• Penetrating wound with difficulty controlling bleeding
• Unconscious
• Signs of shock
  - Lightheadedness
  - Skin that is pale, cold, or moist
  - Thirst
  - Rapid pulse
	Call ambulance immediately.

• Blood is spurting from wound and cannot be controlled with direct pressure. • Exposed bone or deformity at injury site	
• Persistent bleeding > 10 minutes following direct pressure to wound • One or more feminine pad(s) per hour is used. • Gaping bleeding wound • History of bleeding disorder or taking anticoagulant with bleeding • Suspected thrombocytopenia with bleeding	Seek emergency care.
• New bruises without significant trauma • Petechial-appearing rash–little red or purple spots on the skin	Follow homecare instructions. Notify MD if no improvement.

Note. Based on information from Briggs, 2002.

HOMECARE INSTRUCTIONS

To Control Active Bleeding (Friend & Pruett, 2004)

• Stay calm.
• Apply direct pressure for 10–15 minutes. Maintain pressure until bleeding stops. If bandage is saturated, do not remove; apply additional bandages on top.
• Lay patient down and elevate injured part above head (or above heart level).
• Apply ice pack, which helps to control bleeding.

Report the Following Problems

- Swelling/bleeding occurs > 24 hours after bleeding is under control.
- Signs of infection, increased pain, drainage, fever, swelling, pus, streaks or redness.

Suspected Thrombocytopenia Without Bleeding (Friend & Pruett, 2004)

- Avoid trauma, contact sports, or falls.
- Avoid sharp objects or tools.
- Avoid lifting heavy objects.
- Avoid intramuscular injections.
- Avoid medications that contain aspirin or ibuprofen.
- Avoid dental work, floss, toothpicks, and water picks.
- Avoid alcoholic beverages.
- Avoid constipation and enemas.
- Avoid sex, vaginal douches, or tampons if platelet count is < 50,000/mm^3.
- Use an electric razor instead of a razor blade.
- Use a nail file instead of nail clippers.
- Use a soft toothbrush.
- Blow nose gently.

Report the Following Problems

- Blood in urine, vomit, or stool (Friend & Pruett, 2004)
- Prolonged bleeding or bleeding that does not stop

Seek Emergency Care if Any of the Following Occurs

- Signs of shock
- Lightheadedness
- Pale, cold, or moist skin
- Excessive thirst
- Rapid pulse
- Uncontrolled bleeding with suspected thrombocytopenia
- Sudden severe headache, mental confusion, or changes in mood (Friend & Pruett, 2004)

REFERENCES

Briggs, J.K. (2002). *Telephone triage protocols for nurses* (2nd ed.). Philadelphia: Lippincott Williams & Wilkins.

Friend, P.H., & Pruett, J. (2004). Bleeding and thrombotic complications. In C.H. Yarbro, M.H. Frogge, & M. Goodman (Eds.), *Cancer symptom management* (3rd ed., pp. 233–251). Sudbury, MA: Jones and Bartlett.

Lynch, M.P. (2000). Thrombocytopenia. In D. Camp-Sorrell & R.A. Hawkins (Eds.), *Clinical manual for the oncology advanced practice nurse* (pp. 703–707). Pittsburgh, PA: Oncology Nursing Society.

Victoria Wochna Loerzel, MSN, RN, OCN®
Project Director, Breast Cancer Survivor Study
School of Nursing
University of Central Florida
Orlando, FL

Confusion *(change in level of consciousness)*

PROBLEM

No clear or concise definition is used consistently. The patient may not be oriented to person, place, or time, or the patient's behaviors or responses may be inappropriate. A change in level of consciousness can be described as agitation, restlessness, sleepiness, or somnolence, or the patient may be difficult or unable to arouse.

ASSESSMENT CRITERIA

1. What is the cancer diagnosis and treatment?
   Confusion or a change in the level of consciousness can result from multiple causes. These include, but are not limited to, cancer (e.g., glioma, astrocytoma, brain metastasis), cerebral hemorrhage secondary to thrombocytopenia, metabolic disorder (e.g., dehydration), or electrolyte disorder.
2. What medication(s) is the patient taking? Obtain drug history, including over-the-counter medications.
3. Ask patient or family member to describe symptoms in detail.
   a. Is the patient as awake as usual? If not, describe.
   b. Is the patient restless or agitated?
   c. Is the patient confused to time, place, and person or just one or two of these variables?
   d. Is the patient oriented, yet inappropriate?
4. Obtain history, including
   a. Precipitating factors
   b. Onset and duration
   c. Relieving factors
   d. Any associated symptoms, such as headache, recent fall, or seizure.
5. Past medical history
   a. Diabetes mellitus
   b. Cardiac history
6. Changes in activities of daily living

Signs and Symptoms	Action
• Unconscious • Unable to arouse	Seek emergency care. Call ambulance immediately.

(Continued on next page)

(Continued)

Signs and Symptoms	Action

• Seizure
• Altered level of consciousness and any of the following:
  - Severe headache
  - Chest pain/discomfort
  - Rapid heartbeat
  - Diabetic unresponsive to homecare measures
  - Severe abdominal pain
  - Pain worsens on sitting or standing
	Seek emergency care. Call ambulance immediately.

• Altered level of consciousness, arouses, with any of the following:
  - Headache, fever, or stiff and painful neck
  - Recent head injury or trauma
  - Persistent fever
  - Suspected thrombocytopenia
	Seek emergency care.

• New or increased confusion • Change in level of alertness • Mood changes, irritable, tearful, agitated • Change in vision • Loss of movement in limbs • Dizziness • Lethargic • Tremors/shakiness • Not able to get around • Difficulty swallowing	Seek urgent care within 24 hours.
• Sleeplessness • Numbness and tingling (see Paresthesia) • Change in energy level (see Fatigue)	Follow homecare instructions. Notify MD if no improvement.

Cross references: Depressed Mood, Dizziness, Fatigue, Headache, Paresthesia
Note. Based on information from Briggs, 2002.

HOMECARE INSTRUCTIONS

Follow homecare instructions for sleep disturbance, fatigue, or paresthesia as appropriate.

Seek Emergency Care Immediately if Any of the Following Occurs

• Unconscious

- Unable to arouse
- Seizure
- Altered level of consciousness

REFERENCE

Briggs, J.K. (2002). *Telephone triage protocols for nurses* (2nd ed.). Philadelphia: Lippincott Williams & Wilkins.

Margaret Hickey, RN, MSN, MS, OCN®, CORLN

Constipation

PROBLEM

Inability to expel stool or a decrease in usual frequency of bowel movements (Massey, Haylock, & Curtiss, 2004; Tuchmann, 1997)

ASSESSMENT CRITERIA

(Hawkins, 2000; Massey et al., 2004; Tuchmann, 1997)

1. What is the cancer diagnosis and treatment?
   a. Constipation is a common problem in patients with cancer. It is the most common side effect of opioid therapy, and it is a potential problem in individuals receiving neurotoxic chemotherapy, antidepressants, tranquilizers, and muscle relaxants.
   b. It also can be a result of dietary changes, including a decrease in fluid and fiber and a decrease in mobility and exercise. Constipation can be caused by obstruction or compression of the bowel lumen by tumor or ascites. Metabolic changes causing constipation include dehydration, hypokalemia, and hypocalcemia.
2. What medication(s) is the patient taking? Obtain drug history.
3. Ask patient to describe symptoms in detail.
   a. Date of last bowel movement
   b. Was it normal in size, color, and firmness?
   c. Have you had diarrhea?
   d. Was the stool difficult to pass?
4. Obtain history, including
   a. Precipitating factors
   b. Onset and duration
   c. Relieving factors
      i. What have you tried, and what have been the results?
      ii. What have you done in the past if you experienced constipation?
   d. Any associated symptoms.
5. Past medical history (any new medication or treatments)
6. Changes in activities of daily living, including decrease in exercise and activity
7. Dietary history
   a. Decrease in food/fluid consumption
   b. Decrease in dietary fiber

CONSTIPATION

Signs and Symptoms	Action
• Severe abdominal pain, swelling, or vomiting • Vomiting brown, yellow, or green bitter tasting emesis • Significant rectal bleeding with no history of hemorrhoids or bleeding with constipation	Seek emergency care.
• No bowel movement in five to seven days, unresponsive to homecare measures • Recent surgery or injury • History of diverticulitis and fever • Fever for 24–48 hours with unknown cause • Inability to pass gas	Seek urgent care within 24 hours.
• Dry, hard stools • Pain with bowel movements • Recent change in stools or bowel habits • Recent decrease in activity • Recent decrease in dietary intake (fiber) and fluids	Follow homecare instructions. Notify MD if no improvement.

Cross references: Anorexia, Diarrhea
Note. Based on information from Massey et al., 2004; Tuchmann, 1997.

HOMECARE INSTRUCTIONS

(Hawkins, 2000; Massey et al., 2004; Tuchmann, 1997)

- Exercise regularly.
- Drink 8–10 glasses of clear liquid daily.
- Include high-fiber foods in daily diet (exception: caution if taking opioids).
- Drink hot beverages. May drink caffeinated beverages if no other health problems such as high blood pressure or cardiac history.
- Set regular time for daily bowel movement.
- Take stool softeners/laxatives as recommended by physician.

Report the Following Problems (Massey et al., 2004)

- Constipation persists or worsens.
- Homecare measures are ineffective.
- Abdominal pain or cramping
- Vomiting
- Fever

Seek Emergency Care Immediately if Any of the Following Occurs
(Massey et al., 2004)

- Rectal bleeding
- Passing black-tarry stool
- Severe abdominal pain and swelling
- Vomiting brown, yellow, or green bitter-tasting emesis

REFERENCES

Hawkins, R. (2000). Constipation. In D. Camp-Sorrell & R. Hawkins (Eds.), *Clinical manual for the oncology advanced practice nurse* (pp. 339–342). Pittsburgh, PA: Oncology Nursing Society.

Massey, R.L., Haylock, P.J., & Curtiss, C. (2004). Constipation. In C.H. Yarbro, M.H. Frogge, & M. Goodman (Eds.), *Cancer symptom management* (3rd ed., pp. 512–527), Sudbury, MA: Jones and Bartlett.

Tuchmann, L. (1997). Constipation. In R. Gates & R. Fink (Eds.), *Oncology nursing secrets* (pp. 216–225). Philadelphia: Hanley and Belfus.

Kathy Fister, RN, OCN®
Assistant Nurse Manager, Ambulatory Treatment Center
M.D. Anderson Cancer Center Orlando
Orlando, FL

Cough

PROBLEM

A protective reflex used as a defense mechanism by the body to clear airways of secretions and inhaled particles. The term "pathologic cough" refers to a cough resulting from a disease process (McDermott, 2000).

ASSESSMENT CRITERIA

1. What is the cancer diagnosis and treatment?
2. What medication(s) is the patient taking? Obtain drug history.
3. Review past medical and smoking history.
4. Ask patient to describe symptoms in detail, including the presence or absence of sputum production.
5. Obtain history of symptoms, including
   a. Severity
   b. Precipitating factors
   c. Onset and duration
   d. Relieving factors
   e. Any associated symptoms.
6. Changes in activities of daily living

Signs and Symptoms	Action
Are any of the following present? (Attempt to listen to cough and/or breathing over the phone.) • Accessory muscle use • Jugular venous distention • Inspiratory stridor • Expiratory wheezing, crackles, or rhonchi	Seek urgent care within 24 hours.
• Chronic cough (i.e., a cough lasting more than three weeks)	Seek care within one to four weeks if cough is persistent.
Cross reference: Dyspnea *Note.* Based on information from McDermott, 2000.	

HOMECARE INSTRUCTIONS

- Take oral antitussives as prescribed by your healthcare professional.
- Use of a humidifier may be helpful.

Report the Following Problem

- Dyspnea or inability to eat or sleep because of cough

Seek Emergency Care Immediately if Any of the Following Occurs

- Chest pain
- Change in level of consciousness
- Fever
- Sudden increase in dyspnea or dyspnea at rest

REFERENCE

McDermott, M. (2000). Cough. In D. Camp-Sorrell & R.A. Hawkins (Eds.), *Clinical manual for the oncology advanced practice nurse* (pp. 127–130). Pittsburgh, PA: Oncology Nursing Society.

Susan Newton, RN, MS, AOCN®

Deep Venous Thrombosis (DVT)

PROBLEM

A clot that forms in the deep veins, obstructing the flow of blood; emboli may develop.

ASSESSMENT CRITERIA

1. What is the cancer diagnosis and treatment?
   Most commonly seen in patients with cancer of the lung, pancreas, stomach, brain, or colon. Risk factors for deep venous thrombosis (DVT) include sepsis, presence of a venous access device (VAD), cardiac disease, obesity, thrombocytosis, lupus, polycythemia vera, and recent surgery (Lin & Mitchell, 1996).
2. What medication(s) is the patient taking? Obtain drug history.
3. Ask patient to describe symptoms in detail (Story, 2000).
   a. Pain or feeling of tightness in the calf, especially when walking
   b. Vein distention in lower legs
   c. Tenderness over the involved vein
   d. Fever
4. Obtain history, including (Story, 2000)
   a. Precipitating factors
   b. Onset and duration
   c. Relieving factors
   d. Any associated symptoms, such as chest pain and shortness of breath.
5. Past medical history, including previous DVT or cardiac disease
6. Changes in activities of daily living

Signs and Symptoms	Action
• Chest pain or shortness of breath	Seek emergency care. Call ambulance immediately.
• History of the following risk factors: immobility, recent surgery, presence of a VAD, current smoker, infection, active treatment for cancer and diagnosis of cancer of the lung, pancreas, stomach, brain, or colon.	Seek emergency care.

(Continued on next page)

(Continued)

Signs and Symptoms	Action
Past episode of DVT, peripheral vascular disease, recent injury, cellulitis, obstructive lymphadenopathy, or currently on anticoagulant therapy with - Severe pain in the calf of the leg (may or may not be decreased with walking) - Tenderness, warm to touch, redness, or visible blueness or discoloration of any extremity - Fever (low grade) - Palpable vein at tender site - Visible swelling to pitting edema on affected site (or upper arm of VAD site) - Positive Homan's sign (pain on dorsiflexion)	Seek emergency care.
• Any or all of the emergency risk factors listed above with - No shortness of breath or chest pain - Local tenderness with increased discomfort with movement or ambulation - Slight redness or warmth at the affected site - Fever may or may not be present. - Positive Homan's sign may or may not be present.	Seek urgent care within two hours.
• Risk factor of cancer diagnosis and treatment with - A sense of tightness or tenderness in the affected site - No evidence of swelling - Slight warmth in the affected site - Negative Homan's sign	Seek urgent care within 24 hours.
• Any patient who is symptomatic should seek medical evaluation in 24 hours or be contacted for follow-up or current status.	Follow homecare instructions. Notify MD if no improvement.

Note. Based on information from Lin & Mitchell, 1996; Story, 2000.

HOMECARE INSTRUCTIONS

- Elevate leg.
- Reduce ambulation until seen by a physician.
- Do not rub the affected site.
- Do not apply ice or heat unless instructed by the physician.
- Report changes in condition immediately.
- Do not cancel office appointments for any reason.
- Seek medical attention immediately if the symptoms worsen or recur, even if they are in an opposite limb.

Seek Emergency Care Immediately if Any of the Following Occurs

- Shortness of breath
- Chest pain
- Hemoptysis
- Headache
- Unexplained abdominal pain
- Confusion or seizure activity
- Fever with severe pain in an extremity

REFERENCES

Lin, E., & Mitchell, S. (1996). Abnormalities in homeostasis and coagulation. In R. McCorkle, M. Grant, M. Frank-Stromborg, & S. Baird (Eds.), *Cancer nursing: A comprehensive textbook* (2nd ed., pp. 979–1009). Philadelphia: Saunders.

Story, K.S. (2000). Deep vein thrombosis. In D. Camp-Sorrell & R.A. Hawkins (Eds.), *Clinical manual for the oncology advanced practice nurse* (pp. 235–245). Pittsburgh, PA: Oncology Nursing Society.

Mary Murphy, RN, MS, AOCN®, CHPN
Director of Clinical Systems/
Hospice Clinical Nurse Specialist
Hospice of Dayton
Dayton, OH

Depressed Mood

PROBLEM

Feeling sad, disappointed, or upset, which may affect energy level, appetite, and sleep patterns.

ASSESSMENT CRITERIA

1. What is the cancer diagnosis and treatment?
   Recent diagnosis or diagnosis of recurrence, treatment failure, advanced disease stage, unrelieved symptoms (particularly pain), and body image issues that may follow recent disfiguring surgery, such as mastectomy and head and neck surgery, may be associated with depressed mood (Barsevick & Much, 2004).
2. What medication(s) is the patient taking? Obtain drug history.
   Many common medications (e.g., interferon, analgesics, steroids, hormones) prescribed for patients with cancer can have depression as a side effect.
3. Obtain history, including
   a. Precipitating factors
   b. Onset and duration
   c. Relieving factors
   d. Any associated symptoms, such as sadness, teariness, insomnia, change in appetite, change in sleep pattern, and suicidal tendencies.
4. Past medical history
   a. Age (younger people seem to adapt more poorly than older people)
   b. History of depression or substance abuse
      i. Include history of sadness, lasting more than two weeks that was unrelated to illness or a major life event.
      ii. Family history of depression or substance abuse
   c. History of myocardial infarction, surgical procedures
   d. Recent body image changes
   e. Hypothyroidism
   f. Addison's disease, Cushing's disease
   g. Diabetes mellitus
5. Social history (use of alcohol, illicit drugs, and tobacco)
6. Changes in activities of daily living

DEPRESSED MOOD

Signs and Symptoms	Action
A	

• Are five or more of the following signs or symptoms present most of the day, nearly every day during the same two-week period?
  - Loss of interest or pleasure in activities*
  - Depressed mood, feels sad, empty*
  - Hopelessness
  - Insomnia or hypersomnia
  - Significant weight loss or decrease or increase in appetite
  - Psychomotor agitation or retardation (as observed by others)
  - Fatigue or loss of energy
  - Decreased or no interest in sexual activities
  - Feelings of worthlessness or excessive or inappropriate guilt
  - Diminished ability to think or concentrate or indecisiveness
  - Recurrent thoughts of death, suicidal ideation with or without a plan, or suicide attempt or specific plan
	Yes—go to B
	No—go to C

B	

• Not accounted for by
  - Bereavement
  - General medical condition or treatment
	Yes—go to D
	No—go to C

C	
• Are any of the symptoms attributable to side effects of treatment? - Describe signs or symptoms related to treatment (e.g., fatigue, difficulty sleeping, poor appetite).	Yes—refer to triage guideline if available or provide specific homecare instructions to treat symptoms. No—go to D
D	
• Is the patient suicidal? • What plans for suicide does the patient have? • How lethal are the plans? • Is there a gun in the house?	Yes—seek emergency care immediately. No—go to E
E	
• Is the patient currently taking antidepressants?	Yes—continue taking and call prescriber. No—schedule appointment with mental health provider.

*At least one of these has to be present.
Cross reference: Anxiety, Fatigue, Menopausal Symptoms
Note. Based on information from the American Psychiatric Association, 2000.

HOMECARE INSTRUCTIONS

- If treatment is required for depression, it may take weeks to months to notice improvement. Improvement may be seen in
  - Better sleep
  - A decrease in moodiness/grouchiness
  - Ability to focus on tasks
  - Ability to withstand stress without over-reacting
  - Ability to think positively
  - Enjoyment of living.
- Depression can recur. Knowing the symptoms helps to recognize it. Written materials and support groups may be helpful.

Sources for Support Groups and Information

American Cancer Society
www.cancer.org
800-227-2345 (800-ACS-2345)

Cancer Information Service
http://cis.nci.nih.gov
800-422-6237 (800-4-CANCER)

Cancer Care, Inc.
www.cancercare.org
800-813-4673

National Alliance for the Mentally Ill
www.nami.org
703-524-7600 or 888-999-NAMI

National Depressive and Manic Depressive Association
www.ndmda.org
800-826-3632

National Foundation for Depressive Illness
www.depression.org
800-239-1265

National Mental Health Association
www.nmha.org
800-969-6642 (800-969-NMHA)

Department of Health and Human Services
www.hhs.gov
202-619-0257 or 877-696-6775

REFERENCES

American Psychiatric Association. (2000). *Quick reference to the diagnostic criteria from DSM-IV-TR.* Arlington, VA: Author.

Barsevick, A.M., & Much, J.K. (2004). Depression. In C.H. Yarbro, M.H. Frogge, & M. Goodman (Eds.), *Cancer symptom management* (3rd ed., pp. 668–693). Sudbury, MA: Jones and Bartlett.

Mary K. Hughes, MS, RN, CNS
Clinical Nurse Specialist
Psychiatry Section
Neuro-Oncology Department
University of Texas M.D. Anderson Cancer Center
Houston, TX

Diarrhea

PROBLEM

Diarrhea is the passage of loose or watery stools three or more times a day that may or may not cause pain or discomfort in the abdomen and/or rectum (Abramson Cancer Center of the University of Pennsylvania [ACCUP] 2001; Tuchmann, 1997).

ASSESSMENT CRITERIA

(ACCUP, 2001; Engelking, 2004; Tuchmann, 1997)

1. What is the cancer diagnosis and treatment?
   Diarrhea is a common side effect of cancer and cancer therapy, including surgery, chemotherapy, and radiation therapy. Cancers of the gastrointestinal tract (e.g., stomach, colon, rectal) often cause diarrhea. Malignancies that produce hormones can be responsible, such as VIPomas and carcinoid tumors. Chemotherapy drugs affect the lining of the intestinal tract and can induce diarrhea. Radiation therapy causes diarrhea when the area treated includes the abdomen and pelvis. Radiation seed implants for prostate cancer can cause diarrhea. Diarrhea also can be caused by bowel disorders, including Crohn's disease, irritable bowel syndrome, partial bowel obstruction, and bacterial and viral infections, including *Clostridium difficile*. Diarrhea can be secondary to anxiety or nutritional supplement drinks that contain large amounts of vitamins, minerals, sugar, and electrolytes. Patients with constipation may have liquid stool leakage.
2. What medication(s) is the patient taking? Obtain drug history.
   Medications contributing to diarrhea include antibiotics, chemotherapy (5-fluorouracil, irinotecan, interleukin-2), laxatives, diuretics, antihypertensives, antiemetics, sorbitol medications (or foods), magnesium-based antacids, and COX-2 inhibitors.
3. Ask patient to describe symptoms in detail.
   a. Number of stools in 24 hours
   b. Color and consistency of stools
   c. Weight loss
   d. Urine output and character
   e. Signs of dehydration
4. Obtain history, including
   a. Precipitating factors
   b. Onset and duration

   c. Relieving factors

   d. Any associated symptoms, such as abdominal pain/cramps, fever, weight loss, stool incontinence, nausea/vomiting, or decreased urine output.

5. Past medical history
6. Changes in activities of daily living
7. History of bowel habits
   a. Liquid versus formed stool
   b. Color, odor, presence of undigested food or fat
   c. Presence of mucus or blood
8. Diet history
   a. Food intolerance
   b. Aversions
   c. Allergies
9. Social history
   a. Recent travel abroad
   b. Exposure to farm animals or animal feces
   c. Consumption of well water
   d. Ingestion of unpasteurized milk or its products
   e. Consumption of raw seafood

Signs and Symptoms	Action
• Grossly bloody stool • Severe lethargy/weakness • Signs of dehydration • Decreased urine output • Sunken eyes • Pinched skin does not spring back.	Seek emergency care. Call ambulance immediately.
• Excessive thirst, dry mouth • Persistent fever • Diarrhea for more than five days • Seven to nine stools per day with severe cramps • More than 10 stools per day • Weight loss of > 5 lb since diarrhea began	Seek urgent care within 24 hours.
• Less than six stools per day • Chronic diarrhea • Other family members with diarrhea • Recent travel to a foreign country • New prescription	Follow homecare instructions. Notify MD if no improvement.

Cross references: Nausea and Vomiting, Pain
Note. Based on information from ACCUP, 2001; Engelking, 2004; Tuchmann, 1997.

HOMECARE INSTRUCTIONS

(ACCUP, 2001; Engelking, 2004; Tuchmann, 1997)

- Start with clear fluids, broth, and toast.
- Slowly add foods back into your diet, as tolerated.
- Eat a low-residue diet—BRATT: bananas, rice, applesauce, toast, and tea.
- As the diarrhea lessens, add more bland, low-fiber foods, such as boiled white rice, cheese, boiled chicken, and mashed potatoes.
- Eat foods high in protein, calories, and potassium that are easy to digest.
- Eat small, frequent meals. Do not eat large meals.
- Eat foods at room temperature.
- Add nutmeg to foods; this helps to slow down the transition of food through the intestines.
- Avoid milk products.
- Avoid caffeine, alcohol, fiber, dairy, sucrose, sorbitol, olestra, and fried or spicy foods.
- Avoid fresh fruits.
- Cook all vegetables well. Raw vegetables are difficult to digest.
- Avoid greasy, fatty, spicy, or fried foods.
- Refrain from taking fiber supplements.
- Drink plenty of water (at least eight glasses a day) because there is a risk of becoming dehydrated. Sports drinks are helpful because they help to replace electrolytes.
- Do not smoke cigarettes.
- If the diarrhea lasts more than 24 hours, notify your physician.
- Consult your physician before taking any over-the-counter anti-diarrhea medications. These can be very effective but may not be appropriate in your particular situation.
- If prescribed, keep track of medications administered—type, amount, and frequency.
- Clean perineal area well and apply barrier ointment for protection.
- Sitz baths may add comfort.
- Examine rectal area for red, scaly, or broken skin. If present, report to MD.
- Record frequency, quality, and volume of stools during course of treatment.

Report the Following Problems (Engelking, 2004)

- Unable to keep fluids down for 24 hours
- Urine becomes dark yellow in color or no urine
- Dizziness
- Rectal bleeding
- Temperature > 100.4°F
- Swollen and/or painful abdomen
- Red, scaly, or broken skin of the rectal area

Seek Emergency Care Immediately if Any of the Following Occurs
(ACCUP, 2001; Engelking, 2004)

- Severe abdominal pain
- Lethargy/weakness
- Blood and mucus in stools
- Signs of dehydration
- Decreased urine
- Sunken eyes
- Excessive thirst, dry mouth
- Pinched skin does not spring back.

REFERENCES

Abramson Cancer Center of the University of Pennsylvania. (2001, February 11). *Diarrhea.* Retrieved August 9, 2003, from http://www.oncolink.com/treatment/article.cfm?c=2&s=13&id=63

Engelking, C. (2004). Diarrhea. In C.H. Yarbro, M.H. Frogge, & M. Goodman (Eds.), *Cancer symptom management* (3rd ed., pp. 528–557). Sudbury, MA: Jones and Bartlett.

Tuchmann, L. (1997). Diarrhea. In R. Gates & R. Fink (Eds.), *Oncology nursing secrets* (pp. 226–233). Philadelphia: Hanley and Belfus.

Kathy Fister, RN, OCN®
Assistant Nurse Manager, Ambulatory Treatment Center
M.D. Anderson Cancer Center Orlando
Orlando, FL

Difficulty or Pain With Urination

PROBLEM

Difficulty or pain with urination; dysuria

ASSESSMENT CRITERIA

1. What is the cancer diagnosis and treatment?
   Urinary discomfort may be a result of BCG treatment for bladder cancer. Urinary tract infection may cause dysuria, and radiation therapy to the prostate area may result in prostatitis with urinary tract symptoms. Urinary retention can result from spinal cord injury caused by bone metastasis or tumor extension. Hemorrhagic cystitis is a complication associated with ifosfamide and cyclophosphamide.
2. What medication(s) is the patient taking? Obtain drug history.
3. Ask patient to describe symptoms in detail.
   a. Discomfort or pain on urination
   b. Frequency of urination
   c. Feeling that the bladder is emptying fully or not emptying
   d. Time of last urination
4. Obtain history of urinary discomfort, including
   a. Precipitating factors
   b. Onset and duration
   c. Relieving factors
   d. Any associated symptoms, such as blood in urine or fever.
5. Past medical history
   a. Recent urinary catheterization
   b. Sexually transmitted diseases or urinary tract infections
   c. Prostate disease
6. Changes in activities of daily living
7. Sexual practices

Signs and Symptoms	Action
• Urinary retention • Acute flank or back pain • Severe abdominal or groin pain • Temperature > 101.3°F without neutropenia	Seek emergency care.

(Continued on next page)

(Continued)

Signs and Symptoms	Action
• Temperature > 100.4°F with suspected neutropenia	Seek emergency care.
• Hematuria • Dysuria • Burning on urination • Frequent urination—nocturia • Cloudy and/or malodorous urine • Unable to urinate for more than eight hours • Suprapubic tenderness • Flu-like symptoms lasting more than 72 hours • If prior BCG treatment, joint pain, cough, or skin rash	Seek urgent care within 24 hours.
• Recent BCG treatment • Dysuria • Frequent urination • Burning on urination • Difficulty voiding • Slow stream • Dribbling • Sense of incomplete voiding • Urgency • Nocturia	Follow homecare instructions. Notify MD if no improvement.

Cross reference: Fever, Hematuria
Note. Based on information from Aventis Pasteur, 1999; Cope, 2000; Micromedex, Inc., 2000.

HOMECARE INSTRUCTIONS

- Drink 10 eight-ounce glasses of water or more each day (unless contraindicated). Drink cranberry juice, and avoid caffeinated and acidic beverages.
- Cleanse the genital area from front to back and after intercourse.
- Take showers instead of tub baths.
- Monitor urinary output; a voiding diary may be helpful.
- Monitor body temperature every 12 hours and if chills develop.

Seek Emergency Care Immediately if Any of the Following Occurs

- Difficulty breathing
- Loss of consciousness
- Temperature elevation that persists 48–72 hours after treatment

REFERENCES

Aventis Pasteur. (1999). TheraCys® BCG live intravesical. Retrieved February 10, 2004, from http://www.vaccineshoppe.com/US.PDF

Cope, D.G. (2000). Pyelonephritis. In D. Camp-Sorrell & R.A. Hawkins (Eds.), *Clinical manual for the oncology advanced practice nurse* (pp. 567–570). Pittsburgh, PA: Oncology Nursing Society.

Micromedex, Inc. (2000). *Bacillus Calmette-Guérin (BCG) live for cancer (mucosal-local)*. Retrieved December 23, 2002, from http://www.nlm.nih.gov/medlineplus/druginfo/uspdi/202079.html

Denise Dearing, RN, BSN, OCN®
Oncology Nurse Information Specialist
American Cancer Society
Austin, TX

Dizziness

PROBLEM

Dizziness without vertigo can be described as faintness or a sensation of passing out. Dizziness with vertigo includes the sense of either the patient moving or objects moving, often accompanied by nausea and vomiting.

ASSESSMENT CRITERIA

1. What is the cancer diagnosis and treatment?
   Dizziness with vertigo may result from lesions in the inner ear, cranial nerve VIII, brain stem, or cerebral cortex.
2. What medication(s) is the patient taking? Obtain drug history.
3. Ask patient to describe symptoms in detail using specific terms to assist in differentiating between nonvertiginous dizziness and vertigo.
   a. Nonvertiginous dizziness is commonly described as a sensation of the head spinning (light-headed, floating, swimming) while the room remains still.
   b. Vertigo is commonly described as a spinning outside of the head with a sense that the room or patient is moving.
4. Obtain history of dizziness, including
   a. Precipitating factors
   b. Onset and duration (Nonvertiginous dizziness tends to be continuous, whereas vertigo tends to be episodic.)
   c. Relieving factors
   d. Associated symptoms such as tinnitus, hearing loss, positional changes, nausea, vomiting, and diaphoresis.
5. Is there double vision, loss of visual fields, facial numbness or droop, or trouble moving one side (hemiparesis)?
6. Does anything make it better or worse?
7. Does patient have a history of cardiac or vascular disease, diabetes, or blood sugar abnormalities?
8. Does patient have a history of recent upper respiratory infection or ear infections?

Signs and Symptoms	Action
• Chest pain • Difficulty breathing	Seek emergency care. Call ambulance immediately.

(Continued on next page)

(Continued)

Signs and Symptoms	Action
• Incontinence of bowel or bladder • Hemiparesis • Facial numbness • Double vision, loss of visual fields	Seek emergency care.
• Nausea or vomiting (unexplained, not secondary to vertigo) • Headache or ear pain • Known diabetic • Evidence of gastrointestinal bleeding • Temperature > 101°F	Seek urgent care within 24 hours.
• Recent chemotherapy, pain medication, or anxiolytic medication • Spinning feeling • Nausea	Follow homecare instructions. Notify MD if no improvement.

Cross references: Dyspnea, Fever, Headache, Nausea and Vomiting
Note. Based on information from Lafferty & Baird, 2001; Maher, 2000.

HOMECARE INSTRUCTIONS

(Lafferty & Baird, 2001)

- If possible, have family member stay with patient experiencing dizziness.
- Have patient sit with legs elevated or lie down.
- If vertigo is positional, move slowly and take safety precautions to avoid falls.
- Do not drive machinery, such as an automobile, until dizziness is gone.
- Report to physician within 72 hours for evaluation if symptom continues.

Seek Emergency Immediately if Any of the Following Occurs

- Change in level of consciousness
- Vomiting
- Difficulty breathing
- Fever

REFERENCES

Lafferty, S., & Baird, M. (2001). *Tele-nurse: Telephone triage protocols.* Clifton Park, NY: Delmar.

Maher, K.E. (2000). Dizziness/vertigo. In D. Camp-Sorrell & R.A. Hawkins (Eds.), *Clinical manual for the oncology advanced practice nurse* (pp. 729–735). Pittsburgh, PA: Oncology Nursing Society.

Denise Dearing, RN, BSN, OCN®
Oncology Nurse Information Specialist
American Cancer Society
Austin, TX

Dysphagia

PROBLEM

Dysphagia is defined as difficulty in swallowing. The sensation of having the inability to pass food and liquids normally has a negative effect on a person's ability to maintain adequate nutritional status and a level of comfort in their social environment and has a significant impact on quality of life (Iwamoto, 1997). An interdisciplinary approach to managing this side effect, which includes the physician, nurse, registered dietitian, and speech/language pathologist, will optimize the patient's plan of care and treatment outcome.

ASSESSMENT CRITERIA

1. What is the cancer diagnosis and treatment?
   Dysphagia can be a functional symptom of a neurologic problem (cerebrovascular accident [CVA]), a primary central nervous system (CNS) tumor, or a side effect of cancer treatment (Iwamoto, 1997). It is one of the most common side effects of radiotherapy in head and neck cancers and is reported concurrently with stomatitis or esophagitis. Dysphagia also has a structural component resulting from direct tumor extension or surgical resection. Dysphagia in cancer and its therapy can have multiple effects (e.g., swallowing difficulties that can result in dehydration, malnutrition, increased fatigue, suppressed immune function) (Iwamoto). The results can cause an increased risk of infection and treatment interruptions, thus decreasing treatment effectiveness and prolonging recovery time.
2. Obtain past medical history (Grant & Kravits, 2000).
   a. CVA, gastroesophageal reflux disease, or pneumonia
   b. Altered nutritional status
   c. Weight loss (more than 5% over one month or more than 10% over six months)
   d. Infections of the oral/pharyngeal/esophageal mucosa
   e. Alcohol/tobacco use
   f. Placement of nasogastric tube or other invasive procedures of the esophagus
   g. Gastrostomy tube or percutaneous endoscopic gastrostomy placement
3. What medication(s) is the patient taking? Obtain drug history.
   Include date of last chemotherapy treatment.

4. Ask the patient to describe symptoms (Iwamoto, 1997).
    a. Early: "lump" in the throat with or without swallowing; always trying to clear throat
    b. Dry throat: "food gets stuck," the need to swallow food several times before it goes down
    c. Burning sensation of the substernal area with or without swallowing
    d. Coughing/choking with foods or liquids leaking from the nose
    e. Difficulty or pain with swallowing
    f. Choking/vomiting as a result of inability to pass food/fluid
    g. History of dysphagia
    h. Precipitating factors: coughing with liquids/choking
    i. Onset and duration: intermittent with mealtimes or continuous (solids versus liquids)
    j. Relieving factors (dietary modifications)
    k. Treatment of oral infections
    l. Current diet and fluid intake
5. Assess for nutritional plan of care.
    High-risk patients should receive a complete nutrition evaluation by a registered dietitian prior to the initiation of therapy and weekly thereafter. Recommendations include calorie and protein requirements, food consistency options, vitamin replacement, and the use of supplements. Assess labs for albumin and prealbumin and transferrin. Recommendations may include enteral support, with the gastrointestinal tract being the preferred method of support.
6. Evaluate patient's nutritional needs, weight history, and pain management needs once or twice a week, at minimum.
7. Consult with speech pathology for evaluation and treatment to decrease risk for muscle atrophy for swallowing and choking. Will teach strategies for safe swallowing.

Signs and Symptoms	Action
• Inability to swallow with increasing pain, swelling, or compromised airway • Choking/vomiting from inability to pass foods/liquids (or aspiration suspected) • Change in level of consciousness • Temperature > 100.4°F; chills with suspected neutropenia	Seek emergency care immediately.
• Increased difficulty swallowing; unable to eat or drink • Increase in vomiting or pain	Seek urgent care within 24 hours.

(Continued on next page)

(Continued)

Signs and Symptoms	Action
• If feeding tube is present, report nausea/vomiting, indigestion, or diarrhea. • Feeding tube becomes clogged or there is redness, pain, swelling, or leakage from the insertion site • Decreased urine output that is cloudy or dark • Dizziness, increased weakness/fatigue	Seek urgent care within 24 hours.
• Lump in throat/sore throat • Difficulty swallowing	Follow homecare instructions.

Cross references: *Esophagitis, Fever, Mucositis*

HOMECARE INSTRUCTIONS

(Yarbro, Frogge, Goodman, & Groenwald, 2000)
- Follow nutrition plan as developed by registered dietitian.
- Follow exercise/safety plan as developed by speech/language pathologist.
- Take medications as directed.
- Sit upright to maximize swallowing.
- Prevent aspiration: remain sitting for 30 minutes after meals; sleep at a 45° angle.
- Take analgesics as ordered for pain relief to improve intake. If swallowing pills becomes difficult, notify healthcare provider. Not all pills can be crushed.
- Do not smoke or use alcohol.
- Avoid mouth rinses that contain alcohol.
- Perform daily mouth care as instructed, including after meals.

Seek Emergency Care if Any of the Following Occurs

- Inability to swallow with increasing pain, swelling, or compromised airway
- Choking/vomiting from inability to pass foods/liquids (or aspiration suspected)
- Change in level of consciousness
- Temperature > 100.4°F; chills with suspected neutropenia

REFERENCES

Grant, M., & Kravits, K. (2000). Symptoms and their impact on nutrition. *Seminars in Oncology Nursing, 16,* 113–121.

Iwamoto, R.R. (1997). Cancers of the head and neck. In K.H. Dow, J.D. Bucholtz, & R.R. Iwamoto (Eds.), *Nursing care in radiation oncology* (2nd ed., pp. 239–260). Philadelphia: Saunders.

Yarbro, C.H., Frogge, M.H., Goodman, M., & Groenwald, S.L. (Eds.). (2000). *Cancer nursing: Principles and practice* (5th ed.). Sudbury, MA: Jones and Bartlett.

Jackie Matthews, RN, MS, AOCN®
Oncology Clinical Nurse Specialist
Miami Valley Hospital
Dayton, OH

Karen Feldmeyer, RD, LD
Registered Licensed Dietitian
Department of Radiation Oncology
Miami Valley Hospital
Dayton, OH

Dyspnea

PROBLEM

Dyspnea is defined as difficult or labored breathing. Dyspnea is a subjective sensation.

ASSESSMENT CRITERIA

1. What is the cancer diagnosis and treatment?
   a. Dyspnea is common in patients with primary or metastatic cancer involving the lungs, including effusions. Numerous other factors contribute to dyspnea: the cancer itself, general debility, cancer treatments, and other concomitant medical conditions. Dyspnea also may result from pericardial effusions and diaphragmatic pressure with severe malignant ascites or gross hepatomegaly.
   b. Dyspnea can result from surgery with decreased lung capacity after pulmonary resection; radiation therapy when the lungs are in the field, resulting in radiation pneumonitis; chemotherapy with potential pulmonary toxicities, such as bleomycin.
2. Obtain past medical history.
   a. Allergies
   b. Bronchitis, pneumonia, upper respiratory infection
   c. Asthma or chronic obstructive pulmonary disease
   d. Heart disease
   e. Anemia
3. What medication(s) is the patient taking? Obtain drug history.
4. Listen to and describe respiratory pattern.
   a. Any signs of cyanosis—circumoral/nail beds?
   b. Ask to speak to patient on the telephone and listen to respirations for evidence of wheezing, rhonchi, or cough.
   c. Evaluate respiratory and pulse rate.
5. Obtain history of dyspnea.
   a. Precipitating factors
   b. Onset and duration (Determine if dyspnea is an acute or chronic event.)
   c. Relieving factors
   d. Any associated symptoms, such as cough—productive or nonproductive—pain, or fever.

6. Assess for any changes in mental status, including changes in level of consciousness, restlessness, and confusion.
7. Assess for changes in activities of daily living.

Signs and Symptoms	Action
• Sudden and unexpected dyspnea without exertion • Chest pain	Seek emergency care. Call ambulance immediately.
• Dyspnea at rest • Chest pain • New onset hemoptysis with frank red blood • Jugular vein distention • Tachypnea • Temperature elevation	Seek emergency care.
• Increasing dyspnea with activity • Wheezing • Peripheral edema • Uncontrollable cough • Productive cough with yellow, green, or blood-tinged sputum	Report to medical care within 24 hours.
• Pleuritic chest pain • Chronic and stable dyspnea	Follow homecare instructions. Notify MD if no improvement.

Cross references: Anxiety, Cough, Deep Venous Thrombosis
Note. Based on information from Henke, 2000; Lafferty & Baird, 2001; McDermott, 2000; Shelton, 2000.

HOMECARE INSTRUCTIONS

- Feeling short of breath can cause anxiety, and anxiety can worsen the feeling, creating a vicious circle.
- Plan your day to lessen activities that increase dyspnea, such as climbing stairs or bending over.
- Avoid things that make breathing worse, such as tobacco smoke, cold air, and humidity.
- Avoid contact with anyone who has signs of respiratory infection (e.g., cold, fever, sneezing, runny nose).
- Upright position lets the lungs expand and exchange oxygen—sitting up during the day is better than lying flat. Standing up and moving increases the ability for lungs to expand.
- Receive respiratory treatments and oxygen, if prescribed as per physician's order.

- Take pain medicine, per physician's order.
- Take temperature daily or if chilling.
- Make sure that urinary output is adequate.
- Take cough suppressants per physician's order.
- Report any change in sputum.

Seek Emergency Care Immediately if Any of the Following Occurs

- Chest pain
- Change in level of consciousness
- Fever
- Sudden increase in dyspnea or dyspnea at rest

REFERENCES

Henke, S.C. (2000). Pleural effusion. In D. Camp-Sorrell & R.A. Hawkins (Eds.), *Clinical manual for the oncology advanced practice nurse* (pp. 161–166). Pittsburgh, PA: Oncology Nursing Society.

Lafferty, S., & Baird, M. (2001). *Tele-nurse: Telephone triage protocols.* Clifton Park, NY: Delmar.

McDermott, M.K. (2000). Dyspnea. In D. Camp-Sorrell & R.A. Hawkins (Eds.), *Clinical manual for the oncology advanced practice nurse* (pp. 131–135). Pittsburgh, PA: Oncology Nursing Society.

Shelton, B.K. (2000). Pericarditis/pericardial effusion/cardiac tamponade. In D. Camp-Sorrell & R.A. Hawkins (Eds.), *Clinical manual for the oncology advanced practice nurse* (pp. 307–316). Pittsburgh, PA: Oncology Nursing Society.

Denise Dearing, RN, BSN, OCN®
Oncology Nurse Information Specialist
American Cancer Society
Austin, TX

Esophagitis

PROBLEM

Esophagitis is an inflammatory response of the mucosal lining of the esophagus. As with oral mucositis, esophagitis can be measured by severity, including erythema, swelling, ulceration, infection, and possible hemorrhage (Camp-Sorrell, 2000). Dysphagia (difficulty swallowing) is a precursor to esophagitis (Iwamoto, 1997). Odynophagia (painful swallowing) is hallmark, resulting in multiple swallowing problems, nutritional deficits, fatigue, and poor quality of life.

ASSESSMENT CRITERIA

1. What is the cancer diagnosis and treatment?
   Esophagitis is common in patients with head and neck cancers, lung cancer, lymphomas of the chest, or other diseases that include the mediastinum. Patients' risk increases if receiving 5-fluorouracil, doxorubicin, or platinum-based therapy (Camp-Sorrell, 2000). Esophagitis from chemotherapy or radiation is reported during the first two weeks of treatment. Combined treatment modalities will increase the severity of this side effect. Esophagitis is a multifactorial symptom; pain and swallowing difficulties can result in dehydration, malnutrition, increased fatigue, and suppressed immune function (Iwamoto, 1997). The results are an increased risk of infection and treatment interruptions, thus decreasing treatment effectiveness and prolonging recovery time.
2. Obtain past medical history (Grant & Kravits, 2000).
   a. History of altered nutritional status
   b. History of weight loss (> 5% over one month or > 10% over six months)
   c. History of oral hygiene regimen
   d. History of alcohol/tobacco use
   e. Placement of nasogastric tube or other invasive procedures of the esophagus
   f. Gastrostomy tube or percutaneous endoscopic gastrostomy placement
3. What medication(s) is the patient taking? Obtain drug history.
   a. Include date of last chemotherapy, as nadir in the presence of esophagitis may predispose the patient to local or systemic infections.
   b. Identify prolonged use of broad-spectrum antibiotics.
   c. Assess for use of proton pump inhibitors and antacids.
4. Ask the patient to describe symptoms (Iwamoto, 1997).

a. "Lump" in the throat with or without swallowing
b. Dry throat—"food gets stuck"
c. Burning sensation of the substernal area with or without swallowing
d. Epigastric pain
e. Difficulty or pain with swallowing
f. Choking/vomiting as a result of food becoming lodged

5. Obtain history of esophagitis.
   a. Precipitating factors
   b. Onset and duration: intermittent with mealtimes or continuous
   c. Relieving factors (topical anesthesia, systemic analgesia, dietary modifications)
   d. Treatment of oral *Candida*
   e. Current diet and fluid intake

6. Assess for nutritional plan of care.
   High-risk patients should receive a complete nutrition evaluation by a registered dietitian prior to the initiation of therapy and weekly thereafter. Recommendations include calorie and protein requirements, food consistency options, vitamin replacement, and the use of supplements. Assess labs for albumin, prealbumin, and transferrin. Recommendations may include enteral support, with the gastrointestinal tract being the preferred method of support.

Signs and Symptoms	Action
• Sudden increase in frank blood with cough • Persistent fever > 100.4°F, chills with suspected neutropenia • Inability to swallow with increasing pain, swelling, or compromised airway • Choking/vomiting from inability to pass foods/liquids • Chest pain • Change in level of consciousness	Seek emergency care. Call ambulance now.
• Oral assessment indicates increase in inflammation, white patches, or coated tongue. • Unable to drink fluids • Decreased urine output that is cloudy or dark • Dizziness, increased weakness/fatigue • Increasing difficulty swallowing/sore throat	Seek urgent care within 24 hours.
• Sore throat/lump in throat • Difficulty swallowing	Follow homecare instructions.

Cross references: Dysphagia, Fever, Mucositis, Nausea and Vomiting

7. Evaluate patient's nutritional needs, weight history, and pain management needs once or twice a week, at minimum.

HOMECARE INSTRUCTIONS

(Camp-Sorrell, 2000)

- Follow nutrition plan as developed by a registered dietitian.
- Increase fluid intake to 2–3 liters/day or as recommended by dietitian.
- Take topical anesthetics as ordered (30 minutes prior to meals).
- Take antacids and proton pump inhibitors as directed.
- Perform daily mouth care as instructed, including after meals.
- Inspect oral cavity daily for changes in inflammation, presence of white/ yellow patches, and/or coating of the tongue.
- Take analgesics as ordered for pain relief to improve intake. Report problems if swallowing pills becomes difficult. Not all pills can be crushed.
- Take temperature daily.
- Do not smoke or use alcohol.
- Avoid mouth rinses that contain alcohol.
- Add humidity to room air and during sleeping to promote moisture (50%– 60% household humidity).

Seek Emergency Care Immediately if Any of the Following Occurs

- Increase in frank blood with cough
- Change in level of consciousness
- Inability to swallow with increasing pain, swelling, or compromised airway
- Persistent fever > 100.4°F; chills with suspected neutropenia

REFERENCES

Camp-Sorrell, D. (2000). Chemotherapy: Toxicity management. In C.H. Yarbro, M.H. Frogge, M. Goodman, & S.L. Groenwald (Eds.), *Cancer nursing: Principles and practice* (5th ed., pp. 444–486). Sudbury, MA: Jones and Bartlett.

Grant, M., & Kravits, K. (2000). Symptoms and their impact on nutrition. *Seminars in Oncology Nursing, 16,* 113–121.

Iwamoto, R.R. (1997). Cancers of the head and neck. In K.H. Dow, J.D. Bucholtz, & R.R. Iwamoto (Eds.), *Nursing care in radiation oncology* (2nd ed., pp. 239–260). Philadelphia: Saunders.

Karen Feldmeyer, RD, LD
Registered Licensed Dietitian
Department of Radiation Oncology
Miami Valley Hospital
Dayton, OH

Jackie Matthews, RN, MS, AOCN®
Oncology Clinical Nurse Specialist
Miami Valley Hospital
Dayton, OH

Fatigue

PROBLEM

Patient's perceived sensation of tiredness (Nail, 2000)

ASSESSMENT CRITERIA

1. What is the cancer diagnosis and treatment?
   Fatigue is a common symptom with multiple etiologies, which include but are not limited to cachexia, the cancer itself, fluid/electrolyte imbalance, hypoxia, pain, anemia, infection, and a side effect of cancer therapy (chemotherapy and radiation) (McDaniels & Rhodes, 2000; Nail, 2000).
2. What medication(s) is the patient taking? Obtain drug history.
   Any medication that can cause a dry mouth also can cause fatigue. Common medications associated with fatigue include analgesics, antihypertensives, and diuretics.
3. What is the past medical history?
   a. Comorbid diseases (McDaniels & Rhodes, 2000)
   b. Depression (McDaniels & Rhodes)
4. What is the family history?
   a. Depression (McDaniels & Rhodes, 2000)
   b. Recent losses
5. Ask patient to describe symptoms in detail, including the impact on activities of daily living (Nail, 2000).
6. Obtain history of presenting symptoms, including
   a. Precipitating factors
   b. Level of fatigue severity on a scale of 1–10 (lowest to greatest level of fatigue) (Nail, 1997, 2004)
   c. Onset and duration
   d. Relieving factors
   e. Any associated symptoms, such as sleep disturbances, continual sadness, loss of appetite (Nail, 2004).

Signs and Symptoms	Action
• Unable to wake up	Seek emergency care. Call ambulance immediately.

(Continued on next page)

(Continued)

Signs and Symptoms	Action
• Severe fatigue that is disabling; patient is bedridden. • Temperature > 100.4°F with suspected neutropenia	Seek emergency care.
• Severe fatigue or loss of ability to perform some activities • Dizziness • Temperature > 100.4°F without suspected neutropenia	Schedule office visit in 24–48 hours.
• Moderate fatigue or difficulty performing some activities of daily living	Follow homecare instructions. Maintain healthy diet; consider consult with nutritionist or rehabilitation.
• Increased fatigue over baseline but not altering daily lifestyle	Follow homecare instructions. Notify MD if no improvement.

Cross reference: Fever
Note. Based on information from Lin, 2001; McDaniels & Rhodes, 2000; Nail, 1997, 2004.

HOMECARE INSTRUCTIONS

(McDaniels & Rhodes, 2000; Nail, 1997, 2000, 2004)
- Prioritize daily schedule; plan activities.
- Balance work with rest periods.
- Perform moderate exercise.
- Practice energy conservation.
- Eat small, frequent meals throughout the day.
- Increase the amount of clear liquids (8–10 12-ounce glasses/day).
- Practice sleep promotion, including
    - Limit caffeine and alcohol intake.
    - Take short naps during the day, if needed, with exercise (ambulation) in between.
    - Go to bed at a regular time.

Report the Following Problems

- Blood in urine or stool
- Weight loss
- Fever
- Inability to perform activities of daily living

Seek Emergency Care Immediately if Any of the Following Occurs

- Fainting
- Unconsciousness
- Fever occurs with suspected neutropenia.

REFERENCES

Lin, E.M. (2001). Laboratory value assessment. In E.M. Lin (Ed.), *Advanced practice in oncology nursing: Case studies and review* (pp. 278–295). Philadelphia: Saunders.

McDaniels, R., & Rhodes, V. (2000). Fatigue. In C.H. Yarbro, M.H. Frogge, M. Goodman, & S.L. Groenwald (Eds.), *Cancer nursing: Principles and practice* (5th ed., pp. 737–753). Sudbury, MA: Jones and Bartlett.

Nail, L. (1997). Fatigue. In R. Gates & R. Fink (Eds.), *Oncology nursing secrets* (pp. 234–239). Philadelphia: Hanley & Belfus.

Nail, L. (2000). Fatigue. In D. Camp-Sorrell & R.A. Hawkins (Eds.), *Clinical manual for the oncology advanced practice nurse* (pp. 933–939). Pittsburgh, PA: Oncology Nursing Society.

Nail, L. (2004). Fatigue. In C.H. Yarbro, M.H. Frogge, & M. Goodman (Eds.), *Cancer symptom management* (3rd ed., pp. 47–61). Sudbury, MA: Jones and Bartlett.

Anne Invernale, RN, BSN
Chief Operating Officer
Empire State PolyPlants, Inc. and Atlantic PolyPlants, Inc.
Co-Founder, Executive Director, and President
Hortus Carus Foundation
New York, NY

Fever With Neutropenia

PROBLEM

Fever in a neutropenic patient is defined as three oral temperatures > 100.4°F in a 24-hour period or one temperature > 101.3°F.

Febrile neutropenia is a potentially life-threatening emergency (Lynch, 2000).

ASSESSMENT CRITERIA

1. What is the cancer diagnosis and treatment?
   The risk of infection is directly related to the degree and length of neutropenia (Bodey, 2000). More than 60% of patients with neutropenia will develop an infection. Neutropenia can be secondary to malignancies that involve bone marrow infiltration, such as in leukemia, and to chemotherapy and radiation therapy. A neutropenic patient cannot mount a normal response to infection, and fever is often a late sign of an infectious process and could be life threatening (Bodey). Mortality rates during the first 48 hours range from 18%–40% (Lynch, 2000).
2. What medication(s) is the patient taking? Obtain drug history.
3. Ask patient to describe symptoms in detail.
   a. Maximum temperature in 24 hours
   b. Evidence of any other signs of infection (symptoms listed below) (Wujcik, 2004)
4. Obtain history, including
   a. Precipitating factors
   b. Onset and duration, including temperature spikes and time that temperature was elevated
   c. Relieving factors, including any antipyretic medications taken prior to the call
   d. Any associated symptoms, such as open lesions or sores that are red, draining, or tender; mucositis; diarrhea; central venous exit site is red, draining, or tender; sore throat; cough; pain or discomfort with urination; or chills (Wujcik, 2004).
5. Past medical history
   a. Exposure to others with upper respiratory infection or flu
      Review patient's latest complete blood count (CBC) and absolute neutrophil count (ANC) and prior CBCs and ANC during other chemotherapy cycles.

b. Most common cause of neutropenia is chemotherapy, and the timing of neutrophil nadir is predictable and can be estimated based on the agent given.

   i. Always identify chemotherapy agents given and when.

   ii. Review patient's prior ANC with prior chemotherapy cycles. This helps to predict degree of neutropenia, as neutropenia typically worsens with each course of therapy if not treated with a growth factor.

6. Changes in activities of daily living

Signs and Symptoms	Action
• Temperature > 100.4°F • Change in mental status: restlessness, irritability, confusion, or somnolence	Seek emergency care. Call ambulance immediately.

• Rapid breathing, difficulty swallowing, or wheezing
• Signs of dehydration
  - Decreased urine output
  - Sunken eyes
  - Excessive thirst, dry mouth
  - Pinched skin does not spring back.
• Signs of shock
  - Lightheadedness
  - Skin that is pale, cold, or moist.
  - Thirst
  - Rapid pulse	

• Signs and symptoms of infection	Seek urgent care within 24 hours.
• Temperature ≤ 100.4°F	Follow homecare instructions. Notify MD if no improvement.
Cross references: Difficulty or Pain With Urination, Fever, Mucositis	

HOMECARE INSTRUCTIONS

(Wujcik, 2004)

• Take your temperature anytime you feel hot or chilled and every four hours.
• Neutropenic precautions if ANC < 1,000/mm³

Neutropenic Precautions (Wujcik, 2004)

• Good personal hygiene, including hand washing after using the bathroom
• Preventive oral care, including brushing your teeth twice daily and flossing daily. Oral rinse with salt water after each meal.
• Avoid crowds and exposure to anyone with signs of infection.

- Do not change cat litter or clean up animal excreta.
- Nothing per rectum
- Use daily stool softeners to avoid constipation.

Report the Following Problems (Wujcik, 2004)

- Temperature $\leq 100.4°F$
- Chills with or without fever
- New cough with or without sputum or worsening cough
- Burning on urination
- Pain at site of port or catheter
- New sore throat or mouth
- Any area with redness or swelling

Seek Emergency Care Immediately if Any of the Following Occurs

- Changes to level of consciousness
- Shortness of breath
- Signs of shock
- Temperature $> 100.4°F$

REFERENCES

Bodey, G.P. (2000). Fever in the neutropenic patient. In M.D. Abeloff, J.O. Armitage, A.S. Lichter, & J.E. Niederhuber (Eds.), *Clinical oncology* (2nd ed., pp. 690–706). New York: Harcourt Brace and Co.

Lynch, M.P. (2000). Neutropenia. In D. Camp-Sorrell & R.A. Hawkins (Eds.), *Clinical manual for the oncology advanced practice nurse* (pp. 693–698). Pittsburgh, PA: Oncology Nursing Society.

Wujcik, D. (2004). Infection. In C.H. Yarbro, M.H. Frogge, & M. Goodman (Eds.), *Cancer symptom management* (3rd ed., pp. 252–275). Sudbury, MA: Jones and Bartlett.

Victoria Wochna Loerzel, MSN, RN, OCN®
Project Director
Breast Cancer Survivor Study
School of Nursing
University of Central Florida
Orlando, FL

Fever Without Neutropenia

PROBLEM

Temperatures one degree or more above normal constitute a fever. For temperature taken using an oral thermometer, normal body temperature is 98.6°F. Fevers can be described as low-grade (temperatures up to 101°F) and high-grade (temperatures of 102°F or greater that are unresponsive to fever-reducing medicine).

ASSESSMENT CRITERIA

1. What is the cancer diagnosis and treatment?
   a. Fever can be associated with a flu-like syndrome, which accompanies biological response modifiers, and usually peaks between 102°–104°F and often spikes after a rigor. Fever also can result from an infection or from the tumor itself.
   b. It is important to rule out possible neutropenia present in the patient. If the patient is currently receiving cancer therapy or is diagnosed with leukemia, suspect neutropenia and follow guideline for Fever With Neutropenia, as a low-grade fever can be a medical emergency.
2. What medication(s) is the patient taking? Obtain drug history.
3. Ask patient to describe symptoms in detail.
   a. Maximum temperature in 24 hours
   b. Evidence of any other signs of infection (symptoms listed below)
4. Obtain history, including
   a. Precipitating factors
   b. Onset and duration, including temperature spikes and time that temperature was elevated.
   c. Relieving factors, including any antipyretic medications taken prior to the call
   d. Any associated symptoms, such as open lesions or sores that are red, draining, or tender; mucositis; diarrhea; central venous exit site is red, draining, or tender; sore throat; cough; pain or discomfort with urination; or chills (Wujcik, 2004).
5. Past medical history (the following place the patient at high risk)
   a. Diabetes
   b. Steroid use
   c. AIDS
   d. Cardiac problems

    e. Liver or kidney disease

    f. Chronic medical conditions

    g. Exposure to others with upper respiratory infection or flu

6. Changes in activities of daily living

Signs and Symptoms	Action

• Change in mental status: restlessness, irritability, confusion, or somnolence
• Signs of dehydration in an elderly or immunocompromised person
  - Decreased urine output
  - Sunken eyes
  - Excessive thirst, dry mouth
  - Pinched skin does not spring back.
• Signs of shock
  - Lightheadedness
  - Skin that is pale, cold, or moist
  - Thirst
  - Rapid pulse
• Temperature > 103°F and unresponsive to fever-reducing measures
• Rapid breathing, difficulty swallowing, or wheezing
	Seek emergency care. Call ambulance immediately.

• Headache, neck stiffness, and/or photophobia • Temperature > 101°F in the high-risk patient, such as patients with HIV, with leukemia, or on steroids • Fever that persists longer than 72 hours with no known cause • Shortness of breath • Cough with green or yellow sputum • Frequent or painful urination • Rash • Earache, sore throat, swollen glands • Recent surgical procedure	Seek urgent care within 24 hours.
• Congestion, sneezing, and body aches • Other family members are ill. • Fever responsive to self-care measures	Follow homecare instructions. Notify MD if no improvement.

Cross references: Difficulty or Pain With Urination, Fever With Neutropenia, Mucositis
Note. Based on information from Briggs, 2002.

HOMECARE INSTRUCTIONS

(Wujcik, 2004)
- Increase fluid intake (unless contraindicated).
- Rest.
- Take usual medications for fever and aches (acetaminophen or ibuprofen) following instructions on label.
- Take a lukewarm sponge bath or bath soak; do NOT use alcohol rubs or alcohol in water soaks.
- Check temperature every two to four hours or following chills. If no improvement, notify physician.

Report the Following (Wujcik, 2004)

- Temperature increases to > 103°F.
- Fever persists more than 24 hours with no known cause.
- Rash
- Frequent urination, blood or pain with urination
- Signs of dehydration
- Abdominal pain

Seek Emergency Care Immediately if Any of the Following Occurs

- Seizure
- Change in level of consciousness
- Difficulty breathing
- Signs of shock

REFERENCES

Briggs, J.K. (2002). *Telephone triage protocols for nurses* (2nd ed.). Philadelphia: Lippincott Williams & Wilkins.
Wujcik, D. (2004). Infection. In C.H. Yarbro, M.H. Frogge, & M. Goodman (Eds.), *Cancer symptom management* (3rd ed., pp. 252–275). Sudbury, MA: Jones and Bartlett.

Margaret Hickey, RN, MSN, MS, OCN®, CORLN

Flu-Like Symptoms

PROBLEM

A cluster of symptoms may include fever, chills, rigors, myalgia, and malaise. Fever results when pyrogens cause an increase in the body's thermoregulatory "set point." Chills and rigors result when muscle contractions generate heat to raise the body temperature to the new higher set point (Battiato & Wheeler, 2000).

ASSESSMENT CRITERIA

1. What is the cancer diagnosis and treatment?
   Verify if the patient is receiving chemotherapy and/or biotherapy and when the last dose was given. Biological response modifiers such as interferon and interleukin frequently cause flu-like symptoms.
2. What medication(s) is the patient taking? Obtain drug history.
3. Ask patient to describe symptoms in detail.
   a. Fever
   b. Chills
   c. Nausea and/or vomiting
   d. Myalgia
   e. Malaise
   f. Diarrhea
   g. Headache
4. Obtain history of flu-like symptoms, including
   a. Precipitating factors
   b. Onset and duration
   c. Relieving factors
   d. Any associated symptoms, including exposure to viruses or illnesses.
5. Past medical history
   a. Heart disease
   b. Lung disease
   c. Diabetes
   d. Anemia
6. Changes in activities of daily living

Signs and Symptoms	Action
• Neutropenic due to chemotherapy with temperature > 100.4°F	Seek emergency care.

(Continued on next page)

(Continued)

Signs and Symptoms	Action
• Temperature > 103°F without suspected neutropenia • Significant change in blood pressure and/or pulse • Change in mental status	Seek emergency care.
• Symptoms are unrelieved by current methods, as described in homecare instructions.	Seek urgent care within 24 hours.
• If flu-like syndrome is expected from the current therapy	Follow homecare instructions. Notify MD if no improvement.

Cross references: Cough, Diarrhea, Fever With Neutropenia, Headache, Myalgia/ Arthralgia, Nausea and Vomiting

HOMECARE INSTRUCTIONS

(Battiato & Wheeler, 2000; Shelton, 2004)

Treat individual symptoms.
- Fever: Acetaminophen if not contraindicated
  - Tepid soaks, ice packs
  - Fluids (water, bouillon, Gatorade®, Pedialyte®)
- Chills: Warm environment, blankets
  - Hot water bottles (use with caution)
- Myalgia/arthralgia: Rest and relaxation
  - Warm or cold packs
- Headache: Analgesics, dark, quiet environment
  - Frontal headaches secondary to sinus congestion, try a decongestant or warmth and steam.
  - Headache in back of head, apply heat and massage.
- Malaise/fatigue: Rest periods and limitation of activities
- Cough and congestion: Antihistamines, cough suppressants (if upper respiratory)

Seek Emergency Care Immediately if Any of the Following Occurs

- Temperature remains elevated > 3 days
- Vomiting
- Seizure activity
- Change in mental status

REFERENCES

Battiato, L.A., & Wheeler, V.S. (2000). Biotherapy. In C.H. Yarbro, M.H. Frogge, M. Goodman, & S.L. Groenwald (Eds.), *Cancer nursing: Principles and practice* (5th ed., pp. 543–579). Sudbury, MA: Jones and Bartlett.

Shelton, B.K. (2004). Flulike syndrome. In C.H. Yarbro, M.H. Frogge, & M. Goodman (Eds.), *Cancer symptom management* (3rd ed., pp. 61–76). Sudbury, MA: Jones and Bartlett.

Nan Lawary, RN, BSN, OCN®

Staff Nurse

Hematology/Oncology Clinic

Department of Veterans Affairs Medical Center

Dayton, OH

Hand-Foot Syndrome/ Palmar-Plantar Erythrodysesthesia

PROBLEM

A cutaneous toxicity involving primarily the palms of the hand and soles of the feet, but it can occur in other areas, especially pressure-prone areas. It is associated with numbness, tingling, pain, pruritus, erythema, and swelling and can lead to ulceration, blistering, and moist desquamation. Some patients may describe it as a rash (Conrad, 2001; Pike, 2001).

ASSESSMENT CRITERIA

1. What is the cancer diagnosis and treatment?
   Hand-foot syndrome (HFS) is a side effect of some chemotherapeutic regimens, including 5-fluorouracil, doxorubicin, capecitabine, and pegylated liposomal doxorubicin. When HFS occurs, a dose reduction or schedule adjustment is in order (Conrad, 2001; Nagore, Insa, & Sanmartin, 2000). Redness of hands and feet with peeling also may result from strep or other infectious or viral processes.
2. What medication(s) is the patient taking? Obtain drug history, including allergies.
3. Ask patient to describe symptoms in detail.
   a. Location
   b. Appearance
   c. Discomfort rated on scale of 1–10
4. Obtain history, including
   a. Precipitating factors
   b. Onset and duration
   c. Relieving factors
   d. Any associated symptoms such as fever, blistering, pain, skin peeling, paresthesias, or dysesthesias.
5. Past medical history
   a. Recent infection
   b. Exposure to infection
6. Changes in activities of daily living

Signs and Symptoms	Action
• Skin changes (redness, warmth, swelling, dryness, blisters, peeling, drainage, odor, itching) with pain interfering with activities of daily living • Presence of tingling and/or numbness • Patient is taking medications at home known to cause HFS • Fever	Stop taking medications known to cause HFS, such as capecitabine. Seek emergency care.
• Skin changes (redness, warmth, swelling, dryness, blisters, peeling, drainage, odor, itching) with pain interfering with activities of daily living • Presence of tingling and/or numbness • Patient is taking medications at home known to cause HFS • No fever	Stop taking medications known to cause HFS, such as capecitabine. Seek urgent care within 24 hours.
• Skin changes (redness, warmth, swelling, dryness, blisters, peeling, drainage, odor, itching) without pain interfering with activities of daily living • No tingling and/or numbness • Patient *is not* taking medications at home known to cause HFS. • Patient *does not* have a fever.	Follow homecare instructions. Notify MD if no improvement.

Cross references: Fever, Pain, Rash

HOMECARE INSTRUCTIONS

(Haisfield-Wolfe & Rund, 2000; Nagore et al., 2000; Otto, 2001; Pike, 2001; Roche, 2000)

- Avoid injury to feet and hands, tight-fitting clothing, pressure or prolonged heat to hands or feet.
- Avoid topical anesthetics or diphenhydramine-containing creams (may exacerbate skin toxicity).
- Take pain medication as directed by physician or nurse, if ordered.
- Apply alcohol-free emollient cream (Udderly Smooth® or Bag Balm®) liberally and frequently to hands and feet if skin is intact.
- Use cold compresses for comfort.
- Elevate extremities to reduce swelling.
- Monitor for and report signs of infection (e.g., increased redness, pain, drainage, odor).

- Practice good personal hygiene, use mild soap, and no rubbing.
- Wear loose clothing.

Report the Following Problems

- Temperature > 100.5°F with or without signs of infection
- Uncontrolled pain
- Drainage or odor from open areas
- Inability to perform normal daily functions
- Sudden or gradual onset of numbness and/or tingling

Seek Emergency Care Immediately if Any of the Following Occurs

- Blister formation, desquamation (peeling of skin: dry or moist), and infectious complications
- Fever if suspected neutropenia (Pike, 2001; Roche, 2000).

REFERENCES

Conrad, K.J. (2001). Cutaneous reactions. In J.M. Yasko (Ed.), *Nursing management of symptoms associated with chemotherapy* (5th ed., pp. 195–196). West Conshohocken, PA: Meniscus Health Communications.

Haisfield-Wolfe, M.E., & Rund, C. (2000). A nursing protocol for the management of perineal-rectal skin alterations [Electronic version]. *Clinical Journal of Oncology Nursing, 4,* 15–21.

Nagore, E., Insa, A., & Sanmartin, O. (2000). Antineoplastic therapy induced palmar plantar erythrodysesthesia (hand-foot) syndrome incidence, recognition, and management. *American Journal of Clinical Dermatology, 1,* 225–234.

Otto, S.E. (2001). Protective mechanisms. In S.E. Otto (Ed.), *Oncology nursing* (4th ed., pp. 917–947). St. Louis, MO: Mosby.

Pike, K. (2001). Clinical challenges: Hand-foot syndrome [Electronic version]. *Oncology Nursing Forum, 28,* 1519–1520.

Roche Laboratories. (2000). Xeloda® (capecitabine) [Package insert]. Nutley, NJ: Author.

Ana Nunez, BSN, RN, OCN®
Staff Nurse
Sister Caritas Cancer Center
Mercy Medical Center
Springfield, MA

Headache

PROBLEM

Acute or chronic pain in the head. May be attributable to but not limited to
- Emergent causes: Increased intracranial pressure, intracranial bleeding, meningitis
- Nonemergent causes: Stress, sinus congestion/infection, flu or flu-like syndrome.

ASSESSMENT CRITERIA

1. What is the cancer diagnosis treatment?
   a. Primary malignancies of the brain (e.g., astrocytomas and glioblastomas) or metastasis to the brain or skull (e.g., leukemia, lymphoma, breast and lung cancer) and complications of malignancy (e.g., CNS infection in neutropenic patients or syndrome of inappropriate antidiuretic hormone secretion [SIADH] in patients with small cell lung cancer) can increase intracranial pressure, causing pain.
   b. Consider chemotherapy agents with platelet toxicity and timing to nadir, and review recent platelet count and trend for evidence of thrombocytopenia.
   c. Consider biological response modifiers (BRMs) contributing to flu-like symptoms (Shelton, 2004).
   d. Consider cranial radiation as a potential contributing factor to increased intracranial pressure.
   e. Consider headache as a side effect of intrathecal therapy.
2. What medication(s) is the patient taking, both prescribed and over-the-counter? Obtain drug history.
   Use of alpha interferon or other BRMs may cause flu-like symptoms, with headache onset within a few hours of BRMs.
3. Ask patient to describe symptoms in detail
   a. How severe is the pain on a scale of 0–10, with 0 being no pain and 10 the worst imaginable pain?
   b. Where is the pain located?
      Retrobulbar headaches may be associated with flu-like symptoms; frontal headaches may be secondary to sinus congestion; those originating in the back of the head or neck may be related to stress and muscle tension.

4. Obtain history, including
   a. Precipitating factors—identify if any trauma, such as a fall or blow to the head, may be associated with the pain.
   b. Onset and duration
   c. Relieving factors
   d. Any associated symptoms, such as nausea, syncope, photophobia, or visual changes; headaches associated with flu-like syndrome are often retrobulbar and associated with photosensitivity (Shelton, 2004).
5. Changes in level of consciousness, orientation, personality, strength, or gait
6. Changes in activities of daily living

Signs and Symptoms	Action
• Headache accompanied by syncope and visual changes • Headache following head trauma • Known or suspected grade IV thrombocytopenia • Sudden severe pain described as "the worst headache I have ever had" • Uncontrolled or labile hypertension • Drowsiness • Change in consciousness, orientation, personality, strength, or gait • Stiff neck and fever	Seek emergency care.
• Headache worse in the morning, not associated with sinus congestion or fullness • Awakens patient from sleep • Pain uncontrolled by current analgesic regimen • Pain interferes with activity.	Seek urgent care within 24 hours.
• Headache with flu-like symptoms • Pain in facial area over sinuses • Pain/soreness of shoulders and neck • History of temporal mandibular joint dysfunction or pain in joint • History of grinding of teeth (bruxism) • Recently stopped drinking coffee, eating chocolate, or smoking	Follow homecare instructions. Notify MD if no improvement.

Cross references: Flu-Like Symptoms, Pain
Note. Based on information from Lafferty & Baird, 2001; Strohl, 2000.

HOMECARE INSTRUCTIONS

(Lafferty & Baird, 2001)

- Observe for any change in overall status.
- Drink clear liquids sparingly until reason for headache is determined.
- Rest in dark, quiet room.
- Apply ice pack or heat, depending on patient preference, to head and neck.
- Take analgesics as per facility protocol.

Seek Emergency Care Immediately if Any of the Following Occurs
(Wilkes, 2004)

- Loss in or altered consciousness, including restlessness and drowsiness
- Vomiting
- Temperature > 101°F
- Seizure activity

REFERENCES

Lafferty S., & Baird, M. (2001). *Tele-nurse: Telephone triage protocols.* Clifton Park, NY: Delmar.

Shelton, B.K. (2004). Flulike syndrome. In C.H. Yarbro, M.H. Frogge, & M. Goodman (Eds.), *Cancer symptom management* (3rd ed., pp. 61–76). Sudbury, MA: Jones and Bartlett.

Strohl, R.A. (2000). Headache. In D. Camp-Sorrell & R.A. Hawkins (Eds.), *Clinical manual for the oncology advanced practice nurse* (pp. 775–781). Pittsburgh, PA: Oncology Nursing Society.

Wilkes, G.M. (2004). Cerebellar syndromes. In C.H. Yarbro, M.H. Frogge, & M. Goodman (Eds.), *Cancer symptom management* (3rd ed., pp. 389–398). Sudbury, MA: Jones and Bartlett.

Denise Dearing, RN, BSN, OCN®
Oncology Nurse Information Specialist
American Cancer Society
Austin, TX

Hematuria

PROBLEM

Blood in the urine

ASSESSMENT CRITERIA

1. What is the cancer diagnosis and treatment?
   Hematuria is commonly associated with bladder cancer and sometimes a drug-induced inflammation of the urothelium. Associated agents include chemotherapy, such as cyclophosphamide, ifosfamide, and BCG, and biologic therapy, including interleukin-2 and leuprolide acetate. Hematuria also can result from radiation therapy to the pelvic area or from invasive procedures, such as catheterization, cystoscopy, and renal or prostate biopsy. Problems with the urinary tract can cause hematuria, including but not limited to urinary tract infection, glomerulonephritis, and kidney stones (Berry, 2004).
2. What medication(s) is the patient taking? Obtain drug history.
3. Ask patient to describe symptoms in detail.
   a. Amount of blood in the urine—describe by color: pink, red, dark red
   b. Frequency of urination
   c. Pattern of urination
4. Obtain history, including
   a. Precipitating factors
   b. Onset and duration
   c. Relieving factors
   d. Any associated symptoms, such as inability to urinate or pain with urination.
5. Past medical history
6. Changes in activities of daily living

Signs and Symptoms	Action
• Potential internal hemorrhage/massive bleeding • Unresponsiveness • Unconsciousness • Skin color is pale or cyanotic responsiveness	Seek emergency care. Call ambulance immediately.

(Continued on next page)

(Continued)

Signs and Symptoms	Action
• Massive bleeding from urinary tract.	Seek emergency care. Call ambulance immediately.
• Persistent bright-red blood or clots in urine • Urinary or clot retention • Temperature > 100.4°F with suspected neutropenia or > 103°F without suspected neutropenia • Decreased or absent urinary output • Dizziness/lightheadedness	Seek emergency care.
• Low-grade fever without suspected neutropenia • Frequent urination • Pain or buring on urination • Retention • Decreased urinary output	Seek urgent care within 24 hours.
• Intermittent burning (associated with decreased fluid intake) • Bladder spasms • Mild hematuria following therapy for bladder cancer or invasive procedure without suspicion of infection • Frequency known to be associated with noninfectious therapy—post-transurethral resection of bladder tumor (TURBT), biopsy, or other procedure	Follow homecare instructions. Notify MD if no improvement.

Cross references: Difficulty or Pain With Urination, Fever, Pain
Note. Based on information from Berry; 2004; Memorial Sloan-Kettering Cancer Center Division of Nursing, 2000; *Nurse Practitioner's Clinical Companion*, 2000.

HOMECARE INSTRUCTIONS

- Increase fluid consumption.
- Reinforce *normal* symptoms (e.g., spasms) to patient that are associated with postsurgical or related procedures or drugs.
- Consult with MD regarding a prescription for antispasmodic medication.
  - Consult with MD regarding urinalysis or urine culture for dysuria and/ or fever.
  - Limit activities and encourage rest.

Report the Following Problems

- Dysuria

- Fever
- Decreased urinary output
- Urinary or clot retention
- Persistent bright-red blood or clots in urine
- Any bleeding not associated with menses or known urinary procedure

Seek Emergency Care Immediately if Any of the Following Occurs

- Unresponsiveness
- Massive bleeding/hemorrhage

REFERENCES

Berry, D.L. (2004). Bladder disturbances. In C.H. Yarbro, M.H. Frogge, & M. Goodman (Eds.), *Cancer symptom management* (3rd ed., pp. 493–511). Sudbury, MA: Jones and Bartlett.

Memorial Sloan-Kettering Cancer Center Division of Nursing. (2000). *Ambulatory care telephone triage and symptom management protocol manual.* New York: Author.

Nurse practitioner's clinical companion. (2000). Philadelphia: Springhouse.

Terri Armen, RN
Research Nurse
Sarcoma Medical Oncology
University of Texas M.D. Anderson Cancer Center
Houston, TX

Hiccups

PROBLEM

Spasm of the glottis and diaphragm resulting in repetitive, spasmodic inspiratory sounds. Frequently caused by gastric distention, alcohol and tobacco use, sudden excitement, or ingestion of carbonated beverages (Dahlin & Goldsmith, 2001).

ASSESSMENT CRITERIA

(Camp-Sorrell, 2000)

1. What is the cancer diagnosis and treatment?
2. What medication(s) is the patient taking? Obtain drug history.
3. Ask patient to describe symptoms in detail.
4. Obtain history, including
   a. Precipitating factors
   b. Onset and duration
   c. Relieving factors
   d. Any associated symptoms.
5. Past medical history
   a. Recent abdominal, thoracic, or neurologic surgery
   b. Recent emotional problems
6. Changes in activities of daily living

Signs and Symptoms	Action

• Respiratory distress
• Aspiration
• Other life-threatening symptoms
  - Difficulty breathing
  - Lips/mouth blue
	Seek emergency care. Call ambulance immediately.

• Unrelenting hiccups for 48 hours or more with associated signs of exhaustion or dyspnea	Seek urgent care within two hours.
• Describe signs and symptoms that require medical evaluation within 24 hours (e.g., hiccups lasting for longer than 24 hours with early signs of fatigue, loss of appetite, insomnia).	Seek urgent care within 24 hours.

(Continued on next page)

(Continued)

Signs and Symptoms	Action
• Describe signs and symptoms that can be managed at home (e.g., hiccups for less than 24 hours, heartburn).	Follow homecare instructions. Notify MD if no improvement.
Cross reference: Dyspnea	

HOMECARE INSTRUCTIONS

(Camp-Sorrell, 2000)

- Nonpharmacologic measures to cease hiccups: Hold breath, swallow teaspoon of granulated sugar, breathe into paper bag, sip ice water, bite a lemon wedge, pull knees to chest.
- Take medicine as ordered by physician.
- Potential orders may include chlorpromazine 25 mg po QID, haloperidol 1–4 mg po TID, simethicone 15–30 cc q 4 hours, and metoclopramide 10 mg q 6 hours. Consider valproic acid, amitriptyline, nifedipine, baclofen, phenytoin, or phrenic nerve block.
- Monitor for exhaustion/fatigue (e.g., insomnia, anorexia/weight loss, depression), and contact physician's office.
- Monitor for acute symptoms (e.g., dyspnea, aspiration) and seek emergency care, as appropriate.

Report the Following Problems

- No improvement and condition worsens
- Suspected side effects from medication

Seek Emergency Care Immediately if Any of the Following Occurs

- Shortness of breath
- Aspiration of food
- Blueness of lips/mouth
- Inability to swallow

REFERENCES

Camp-Sorrell, D. (2000). Hiccups. In D. Camp-Sorrell & R.A. Hawkins (Eds.), *Clinical manual for the oncology advanced practice nurse* (pp. 13–16). Pittsburgh, PA: Oncology Nursing Society.

Dahlin, C., & Goldsmith, T. (2001). Dysphagia, dry mouth and hiccups. In B. Ferrell & N. Coyle (Eds.), *Textbook of palliative nursing* (pp. 122–138). New York: Oxford University Press.

Christy Erikson, RN, MSN, NP, AOCN®
Nurse Practitioner, Hematology/Oncology Clinic
Fletcher Allen Health Care
Burlington, VT

Lymphedema

PROBLEM

An accumulation of lymph fluid in the interstitial spaces caused by an increase in production of lymph fluid or an obstruction of the lymphatic drainage system. Primary lymphedema occurs with no obvious etiology. Secondary lymphedema is caused by injury, scarring, or removal of the lymph nodes (National Lymphedema Network, 2004).

ASSESSMENT CRITERIA

1. What is the cancer diagnosis and treatment? Was a lymph node dissection performed? What site is affected?
   The most common sites of obstruction are the pelvic, inguinal, and axillary nodes.
2. What medication(s) is the patient taking? Obtain drug history.
3. Review past medical history and activities prior to occurences of lymphedema.
4. Ask patient to describe symptoms in detail, such as pain, onset and extent of edema, skin changes, exercise patterns, and range of motion.
5. Obtain history of symptoms, including
   a. Severity
   b. Precipitating factors: May occur after an injury, infection, excessive physical exertion, or airplane travel.
   c. Onset and duration: Onset may be sudden or gradual.
   d. Relieving factors
   e. Any associated symptoms
   f. Risk factors, including lymph node dissection, radiation therapy to areas of lymph nodes, infections, obesity, and age
6. Changes in activities of daily living

Signs and Symptoms	Action
• Red streaks going up and down the limb • Pain or soreness that is in one area or came on suddenly • Swelling	Seek urgent care within 24–48 hours.
• Sudden increase in edema in an extremity • Tightness of clothing or rings, numbness or pain	Seek care within one week.
Cross reference: Deep Venous Thrombosis *Note.* Based on information from Cope, 2000.	

LYMPHEDEMA

HOMECARE INSTRUCTIONS

(Kalinowski, 2004; Saskia & Thiadens, 2002)

Lymphedema can develop in any part of the body or limb(s).

- Signs or symptoms of lymphedema to watch for include a full sensation in the limb(s); skin feeling tight; decreased flexibility in the hand, wrist, or ankle; difficulty fitting into clothing in one specific area; or ring/wristwatch/bracelet tightness.
- Patients who have undergone lymph node dissections always should avoid blood draws, injections, IV placement, and blood pressure monitoring in the affected extremity. Use extra precautions to avoid injury to the affected extremity.
- Planning the treatment program depends on the cause of the lymphedema. For example, if the initial signs and symptoms of swelling are caused by infection (redness, rash, heat, blister, or pain), antibiotics will need to be prescribed first. Treating an infection often reduces some of the swelling and discoloration.
- If the lymphedema is not caused by infection, depending on the severity of the lymphedema, the recommended treatment plan should be determined using an approach based on the complex decongestive therapy methods. These consist of (a) manual lymphatic drainage, (b) bandaging, (c) proper skin care and diet, (d) compression garments (e.g., sleeves, stockings), (e) remedial exercises, (f) self-manual lymphatic drainage and bandaging, and (g) the continual use of prophylactic methods at all times.

Report the Following Problems Promptly

- Redness or areas of skin irritation or breakdown (suspect cellulitis)
- Sudden onset of severe pain, tenderness, area is warm to touch, obvious blueness or other discoloration, increased pain with dorsiflexion (suspect deep vein thrombosis) (Cope, 2000)

REFERENCES

Cope, D. (2000). Lymphedema. In D. Camp-Sorrell & R.A. Hawkins (Eds.), *Clinical manual for the oncology advanced practice nurse* (pp. 649–652). Pittsburgh, PA: Oncology Nursing Society.
Kalinowski, B.H. (2004). Lymphedema. In C.H. Yarbro, M.H. Frogge, & M. Goodman (Eds.), *Cancer symptom management* (3rd ed., pp. 461–474). Sudbury, MA: Jones and Bartlett.
National Lymphedema Network. (2004). *Lymphedema: A brief overview.* Retrieved July 8, 2003, from http://www.lymphnet.org/whatis.html
Saskia, R.J., & Thiadens, R.N. (2002). *Lymphoma: An information booklet.* Oakland, CA: National Lymphoma Network.

Susan Newton, RN, MS, AOCN®

Menopausal Symptoms

PROBLEM

Menopause is the end of menstruation for at least 12 months as the result of the loss of ovarian function (Cormier, 2000). Menopausal symptoms are a cluster of physical and psychological events women experience when there is a shift in estrogen (Moore, 2004).

ASSESSMENT CRITERIA

(Cormier, 2000)

1. What is the cancer diagnosis and treatment?
   Pelvic radiation, oophorectomy, and certain chemotherapy agents place a woman at risk for early menopause.
2. What medication(s) is the patient taking? Obtain drug history.
3. Review past medical history.
4. Ask patient to describe symptoms in detail.
5. Obtain history of symptoms, including
   a. Severity
   b. Precipitating factors
   c. Onset and duration
   d. Relieving factors
   e. Any associated symptoms, such as hot flashes, night sweats, and insomnia
6. Changes in activities of daily living

Signs and Symptoms	Action
• Chest pain or shortness of breath	Seek emergency care. Call ambulance immediately.
• Severe headache • Pain in calf (women on hormone therapy or estrogen replacement therapy) • Heavy vaginal bleeding present (soaking more than one pad an hour or bleeding accompanied by weakness or dizziness)	Seek emergency care.

(Continued on next page)

(Continued)

Signs and Symptoms	Action
• Panic attacks, self-destructive behavior, delirium or disorientation, suicidal ideation or plan, or any life-threatening symptoms	Seek emergency care.
• Breast lump or tenderness • Postmenopausal vaginal bleeding • Persistent nausea, vomiting	Seek urgent care within 24 hours.
• Sleep disruption • Vaginal discharge • Mood changes, difficulty making decisions • Hot flashes and night sweats • Vaginal dryness or itching • Headaches	Follow homecare instructions. Notify MD if no improvement.

Cross reference: Anxiety, Bleeding, Depressed Mood, Deep Venous Thrombosis, Headache
Note. Based on information from Cormier, 2000; Love, 1997; Moore, 2004.

HOMECARE INSTRUCTIONS

Hot Flashes (Asch-Goodkin, 2001; Cormier, 2000; Love, 1997; Moore, 2004; Northrup, 1998)

• Keep a diary of menopausal symptoms. This diary can be used to help to identify triggers for hot flashes. Common triggers include hot drinks, caffeine, alcohol, spicy foods, stress, and smoking.
• Lower your thermostat; use fans and air conditioning.
• Dress in layers.
• Wear absorbent clothing, such as cotton. Avoid wool and synthetics.
• Keep a glass of ice water on hand.
• Talk to your healthcare provider about over-the-counter remedies. Many herbal products contain estrogen-like substances that may be contraindicated in patients with hormone-sensitive tumors.

Vaginal Dryness (Cormier, 2000; Love, 1999; Moore, 2004)

• Warm baths may help to relieve itching and discomfort.
• Avoid douches or feminine hygiene sprays.
• Use nonperfumed soaps and toilet paper.
• Try over-the-counter vaginal lubricants or moisturizers.

Insomnia (Asch-Goodkin, 2001; Cormier, 2000; Love, 1997; Moore, 2004)
- Practice regular aerobic exercise.
- Practice relaxation techniques (e.g., yoga, deep breathing, meditation).
- Avoid alcohol and caffeine.
- Keep a regular bedtime schedule and routine.
- Eat a light dinner.

Seek Emergency Care Immediately if Any of the Following Occurs
(Love, 1997; Moore, 2004)
- Chest pain
- Severe dyspnea
- Calf pain (women taking hormone or estrogen-replacement therapy)
- Hemoptysis
- Severe headache
- Severe vaginal bleeding
- Suicidal ideation

REFERENCES

Asch-Goodkin, J. (2001, May). Caring for the post-menopausal woman: Complete care of the older woman. *Patient Care for the Nurse Practitioner, 5,* 15–27.

Cormier, A.C. (2000). Menopausal symptoms and menopause. In D. Camp-Sorrell & R.A. Hawkins (Eds.), *Clinical manual for the oncology advanced practice nurse* (pp. 903–925). Pittsburgh, PA: Oncology Nursing Society.

Love, S. (1997). *Dr. Susan Love's hormone book.* New York: Random House.

Moore, S. (2004). Menopausal symptoms. In C.H. Yarbro, M.H. Frogge, & M. Goodman (Eds.), *Cancer symptom management* (3rd ed., pp. 571–595). Sudbury, MA: Jones and Bartlett.

Northrup, C. (1998). *Women's bodies, women's wisdom.* New York: Bantam Books.

Shirley Williams, RN, CS, AOCN®
Consultant
Port Townsend, WA

Rita Mahaffey, RN, BSN, OCN®
Breast Care Coordinator
M.D. Anderson Cancer Center Orlando
Orlando, FL

Rae M. Norrod, MS, RN, AOCN®
Clinical Nurse Specialist
Kettering Medical Center Network
Kettering, OH

Carol Pilgrim, APRN, BC
Nurse Practitioner
Carle Clinic Association
Urbana, IL

Mucositis

PROBLEM

Inflammation of the mucous membranes commonly occurring in the oral cavity

ASSESSMENT CRITERIA

(Kemp & Brackett, 1997; Strohl, 2000)

1. What is the cancer diagnosis and treatment?
   Mucositis can develop as a side effect of a variety of chemotherapy agents within 5–7 days of administration, radiation therapy to the oral cavity within 7–10 days, bone marrow transplantation, recent oral surgery, or poor oral hygiene. Xerostomia, or dryness of the oral cavity, contributes to the development of mucositis. The mouth is the most frequently documented source of infection in immunocompromised patients.
2. What medication(s) is the patient taking? Obtain drug history.
3. Ask patient to describe symptoms in detail.
   a. Location of erythema, ulceration, and/or pain
   b. Erythema of mouth, gums, cheeks, and tongue
   c. Ulceration
   d. Any white patches (cottage cheese–like patches)
   e. Xerostomia
   f. Pain
   g. Difficulty with swallowing
   h. Hoarseness
   i. Fever
4. Obtain history, including
   a. Past medical history of HIV
   b. History of nutritional intake, current diet, weight loss, and current oral hygiene practices
   c. Social history of tobacco and/or alcohol use.
5. Assessment
   a. Location
      i. Lips
      ii. Gums
      iii. Buccal mucosa
      iv. Tongue
      v. Soft palate
   b. Characteristics

      i. Erythema
     ii. Blisters
   iii. Ulcers
   iv. White patches
  c. Precipitating factors
      i. Pain or discomfort all of the time
     ii. Pain or discomfort only with oral intake
  d. Onset and duration
      i. Chronic or only with oral intake
     ii. Condition stable or worsening
  e. Relieving factors
      i. Ice chips
     ii. Local or systemic analgesics
  f. Any associated symptoms such as fever, decreased oral intake, sore throat, dysphagia, vaginal symptoms

6. Changes in activities of daily living

Signs and Symptoms	Action
• Severe ulceration and unable to take po (intake < 500 ml/24 hours) • Bleeding that will not stop • Temperature > 100.4°F with suspected neutropenia	Seek emergency care.
• Painful erythema, edema, or ulcers that prevent swallowing • Signs of dehydration • Decreased urine • Sunken eyes • Pinched skin does not spring back. • Excessive thirst, dry mouth • Oral intake < 1,000 ml/24 hours • White, cottage cheese–like patches in the mouth • Oral bleeding • Fever • Pain unrelieved by homecare measures rated > 3 on scale of 1–10 • Inability to eat soft foods	Seek urgent care within 24 hours.
• Painful erythema, edema, or ulcer and still able to eat and swallow • Painless ulcer, erythema, or mild soreness without lesions • Mild pain rated < 3 on scale 1–10	Follow homecare instructions. Notify MD if no improvement.

Cross references: Bleeding, Dysphagia, Esophagitis, Fever, Pain, Xerostomia
Note. Based on information from Kemp & Brackett, 1997.

HOMECARE INSTRUCTIONS

(Beck, 2004; Kemp & Brackett, 1997)

- Inspect mouth daily and call if changes occur.
- Use a water-based mouth moisturizer.
- Practice good oral hygiene.
- Use soft toothbrush and brush teeth TID.
- Mouth rinses with salt water, 2 tsp. in quart of warm water, or salt and soda rinses with 1 tsp. each in a quart of warm water, four times daily. Increase frequency until it is given every hour while awake and every four hours at night when mouth becomes painful and ulcers are present.
- Avoid commercial mouthwashes, as they contain alcohol.
- If prescribed, use swish and swallow solutions.
- Remove dentures, except to eat; keep them clean; soak them in baking soda.
- Avoid alcoholic beverages.
- Avoid spicy, acidic foods.
- Avoid tobacco smoking.
- Increase fluid intake > 1,500 ml/24 hours unless contraindicated.
- Follow a high-protein diet.

Report the Following Problems (Beck, 2004; Strohl, 2000)

- Oral intake > 1 liter/24 hours
- Mouth sores starting to develop
- Pain rated > 5 on a 1–10 scale
- Foul odor from mouth
- Worsening of symptoms
- Fever
- Bleeding from gums, oral cavity, or mouth

Seek Emergency Care Immediately if Any of the Following Occurs

- Inability to drink or swallow
- Uncontrolled bleeding
- Difficulty breathing
- Continued temperature > 100.4°F not controlled with acetaminophen and previously prescribed antibiotics (Beck, 2004).

REFERENCES

Beck, S.L. (2004). Mucositis. In C.H. Yarbro, M.H. Frogge, & M. Goodman (Eds.), *Cancer symptom management* (3rd ed., pp. 276–292). Sudbury, MA: Jones and Bartlett.

Kemp, J., & Brackett, H. (1997). Mucositis. In R. Gates & R. Fink (Eds.), *Oncology nursing secrets* (pp. 245–261). Philadelphia: Hanley and Belfus.

Strohl, R. (2000). Stomatitis/xerostomia. In D. Camp-Sorrell & R.A. Hawkins (Eds.), *Clinical manual for the oncology advanced practice nurse* (pp. 63–66). Pittsburgh, PA: Oncology Nursing Society.

Dolores Tanner, RN, OCN®
Medical Oncology Outpatient Nurse
M.D. Anderson Cancer Center Orlando
Orlando, FL

Lisa Feldsien, RN, BSN, OCN®
Staff Nurse
Western Baptist Hospital
Paducah, KY

Nancy Lange, RN, OCN®
Weekend Telephone Triage Nurse
Cancer Care Associates
Oklahoma City, OK

Myalgia/Arthralgia ("hurts all over")

PROBLEM

Generalized muscle and joint pains: Tissue damage causes the release of brady-kinin, which stimulates muscle nociceptors.

ASSESSMENT CRITERIA

1. What is the cancer diagnosis and treatment?
   Arthralgia and myalgia can be caused by a number of factors, including chemotherapy and biotherapy. A contributing list of potential causes for diffuse arthralgia and myalgia is as follows.
   a. Drug-induced—chemotherapy agents including taxanes (paclitaxel/docetaxel), biotherapy (interferon, interleukin), colony-stimulating growth factors, and some antibiotics (Martin, 2004; Shelton, 2004; Verstappen, Heimans, & Postma, 2003).
   b. Infectious—influenza or intercurrent viral or viral-like syndromes, HIV, dengue fever, Lyme disease, cytomegalovirus syndrome
   c. Overuse syndromes
   d. Endocrine/metabolic—prolonged or sudden withdrawal of corticosteroid therapy; electrolyte disturbances; diabetes mellitus
   e. Autoimmune
   f. Neoplastic/hematologic—initial presentation of certain malignancies (e.g., lymphoma, leukemia) or paraneoplastic syndromes (Ferri, 2003)
   g. Psychiatric—stress, anxiety, tension
   h. Other—fibromyalgia, chronic fatigue syndrome, silicone implant syndrome (most have fibromyalgia), vasculitis (Collins, 2003)
2. What medication(s) is the patient taking? Obtain drug history.
3. Ask patient to describe symptoms in detail.
   a. Fever
   b. Chills
   c. Edema
   d. Fatigue
   e. Headache
4. Obtain history, including
   a. Precipitating factors
   b. Onset and duration
   c. Relieving factors
   d. Any associated symptoms, such as fever.

5. Past medical history (fibromyalgia)
6. Changes in activities of daily living

Signs and Symptoms	Action
• Acute injury, paralysis, pending respiratory failure, or other life-threatening symptoms, including - Sudden onset of severe, unrelenting pain - Inability to ambulate - Extremity or joint swelling with chest pain - Acute joint deformity • Difficulty breathing • Cyanosis—skin, extremity, or lips turning blue	Seek emergency care. Call ambulance immediately.
• Temperature > 100.4°F associated with recent chemotherapy treatment • Recent onset of neurologic manifestations • New or sudden onset of inability to ambulate or bear weight • Unexplained difficulty in or rapid breathing • Swelling in one extremity and a recent history of immobility or a history of blood clots in legs • Jaundice and dark urine	Seek urgent care within two hours.
• Progressive symptoms associated with temperature > 100.4°F • Unexplained symptoms associated with patient history of bone marrow or organ transplant, recent dental or surgical procedure, recent history of travel to tropical areas within two weeks of the onset of symptoms • Constitutional symptoms (symptom indicating a systemic effect of a disease) (e.g., weight loss, night sweats, anorexia, general malaise) • New headache • Diffuse muscular weakness • Recent history of insect or tick bite associated with - Visual symptoms - Bilateral symptoms - Claudication	Seek urgent care within 24 hours. (Consider consultation with infectious disease specialist, neurologist, rheumatologist, or endocrinologist, as indicated.)

(Continued on next page)

(Continued)

Signs and Symptoms	Action
- Rash - Regional and generalized lymphadenopathy or other unexplained localized joint redness, swelling, or hyperthermia - New prescription medicine	Seek care within 24 hours. (Consider consultation with infectious disease specialist, neurologist, rheumatologist, or endocrinologist, as indicated.)
• Recent onset *without* fever or with low-grade fever and nonprogressive symptoms • Onset to symptoms is associated with intercurrent viral or viral-like syndrome. • Onset to symptoms is drug induced, such as chemotherapy agents (including taxanes), biologic agents (including interferon, interleukin, hematopoietic growth factors, and immunotoxin), or the recent withdrawal of corticosteroids (including dexamethasone or prednisone). • Symptoms associated with recent extensive physical workout	Follow homecare instructions. Notify MD if no improvement. Consult with MD regarding tapering of corticosteroids as indicated.

Cross references: Fever, Flu-Like Symptoms, Headache, Nausea and Vomiting
Note. Based on information from Christian, 1994; Wilkes, Ingwersen, & Barton-Burke, 2002.

HOMECARE INSTRUCTIONS

- Increase fluid consumption.
- As recommended by physician, and if not contraindicated, take acetaminophen, aspirin, ibuprofen, or other analgesics as prescribed per label instructions for fever and generalized achiness (Martin, 2004; Shelton, 2004).
- Limit activity; rest.
- Additional instructions: treat symptomatically.

Report the Following Problems

- No improvement or condition worsens
- Fever that persists for 24 hours with unknown cause
- Symptoms are progressive or persistent (more than one week)
- Increasing pain unrelieved by acetaminophen or ibuprofen as recommended by the physician

Seek Emergency Care Immediately if Any of the Following Occurs

- Chest pain
- Unresponsiveness
- Difficulty breathing

REFERENCES

Christian, C.L. (1994). Musculoskelatal syndromes. In J.A. Barondess, C.J. Carpenter, & A.M. Harvey (Eds.), *Differential diagnosis* (pp. 811–841). Philadelphia: Lea & Febiger.

Collins, R.D. (2003). *Differential diagnosis in primary care* (3rd ed.). Philadelphia: Lippincott Williams & Wilkins.

Ferri, F.F. (2003). *Ferri's clinical advisor–instant diagnosis and treatment*. St. Louis, MO: Mosby.

Martin, V.R. (2004). Arthralgias and myalgias. In C.H. Yarbro, M.H. Frogge, & M. Goodman (Eds.), *Cancer symptom management* (3rd ed., pp. 17–28). Sudbury, MA: Jones and Bartlett.

Shelton, B.K. (2004). Flulike syndrome. In C.H. Yarbro, M.H. Frogge, & M. Goodman (Eds.), *Cancer symptom management* (3rd ed., pp. 61–76). Sudbury, MA: Jones and Bartlett.

Verstappen, C., Heimans, K.H., & Postma, T.J. (2003). Neurotoxic complications of chemotherapy in patients with cancer: Clinical signs and optimal management. *Drugs, 63,* 1549–1563.

Wilkes, G.M., Ingwersen, K., & Barton-Burke, M. (2002). *2002 oncology nursing drug handbook.* Sudbury, MA: Jones and Bartlett.

Lori Lindsey, RNC, FNP, OCN®
Nurse Practitioner
Texas Cancer Associates
Dallas, TX

Nausea and Vomiting

PROBLEM

Nausea is an unpleasant sensation described as the need to vomit or queasiness that may occur before, with, or without vomiting (Murphy-Ende, 2000). Vomiting is the expulsion of gastric contents through the mouth (Murphy-Ende).

ASSESSMENT CRITERIA

(Camp-Sorrell, 2000; Murphy-Ende, 2000; Wickham, 2004)

1. What is the cancer diagnosis and treatment?
   The causes of nausea and vomiting can be therapy-related (chemotherapy and radiation therapy) or related to the disease.
2. What medication(s) is the patient taking? Obtain drug history.
3. Ask patient to describe symptoms in detail.
   a. Nausea with or without vomiting
   b. Any frank blood or coffee-ground emesis
   c. Oral intake of food and liquids
   d. Urinary frequency
   e. Constipation
   f. Pain
   g. Viral symptoms such as malaise, myalgia, arthralgia, headache, fever, rhinitis, or cough (or family member with these symptoms)
4. Obtain history of nausea and vomiting, including
   a. Precipitating factors
   b. Onset and duration
      i. Frequency of vomiting episode(s)
      ii. Length of time nausea and/or vomiting has been occurring
   c. Relieving factors
   d. Any associated symptoms, such as increased salivation, diaphoresis, tachycardia, diarrhea, retching, dysphagia, and thirst
5. Past medical history, including family history

Signs and Symptoms	Action
• Chest pain, difficulty breathing, palpitations, or sweating	Seek emergency care.

(Continued on next page)

(Continued)

Signs and Symptoms	Action
• Decreased level of consciousness • Fainting • Recent injury to head or abdomen and vomiting • Blood or coffee-ground-appearing material in emesis • Severe stomach pain while vomiting	Seek emergency care.
• Nausea with no significant intake for more than 24 hours • Vomiting > six episodes in 24 hours • Projectile vomiting • Weakness, dizziness along with nausea/vomiting • Temperature > 100.4°F with suspected neutropenia • Nausea and vomiting persisting after 24 hours with antiemetic therapy	Seek urgent care within 24 hours.
• Nausea but able to eat • Vomiting, one episode in 24 hours • Diarrhea or constipation • Other household members who have been or are ill • Recent addition of antibiotic, analgesic, or other new medication	Follow homecare instructions. Notify MD if no improvement.

Cross references: Anorexia, Fever
Note. Based on information from Camp-Sorrell, 2000; Murphy-Ende, 2000; Wickham, 2004.

HOMECARE INSTRUCTIONS

(Camp-Sorrell, 2000; Murphy-Ende, 2000; Wickham, 2004)

- Drink clear fluids; no caffeine.
- Eat bland foods; no spicy/fried foods.
- May try products with ginger/lemon.
- Avoid odors and stress when eating.
- Eat and drink slowly.
- Eat small, frequent meals throughout the day.
- Use distraction techniques.
- Continue good mouth care.
- May try acupressure.
- Continue or begin antiemetics as prescribed by physician.

Report the Following Problems (Wickham, 2004)

- Headache
- Dizziness
- Back pain
- Tinnitus
- Jaundice, itching
- Abdominal pain, swelling, heartburn
- Temperature > 100.4°F
- Coffee-ground emesis

Seek Emergency Care Immediately if Any of the Following Occurs
(Wickham, 2004)

- Sudden projectile vomiting
- Blurred vision
- Confusion

REFERENCES

Camp-Sorrell, D. (2000). Chemotherapy: Toxicity management. In C.H. Yarbro, M.H. Frogge, M. Goodman, & S.L. Groenwald (Eds.), *Cancer nursing: Principles and practice* (5th ed., pp. 456–463). Sudbury, MA: Jones and Bartlett.

Murphy-Ende, K. (2000). Nausea and vomiting. In D. Camp-Sorrell & R.A. Hawkins (Eds.), *Clinical manual for the oncology advanced practice nurse* (pp. 379–385). Pittsburgh, PA: Oncology Nursing Society.

Wickham, R. (2004). Nausea and vomiting. In C.H. Yarbro, M.H. Frogge, & M. Goodman (Eds.), *Cancer symptom management* (3rd ed., pp. 187–214). Sudbury, MA: Jones and Bartlett.

Kimberly Morrison, BSN, MN, AOCN®, ARNP
Oncology Nurse Practitioner
M.D. Anderson Cancer Center Orlando
Orlando, FL

Pain

PROBLEM

An unpleasant sensation caused by actual or potential tissue damage (Thomas, 1997)

ASSESSMENT CRITERIA

1. What is the cancer diagnosis and treatment?
   Pain is experienced by nearly one-third of patients receiving treatment for cancer and two-thirds of patients with advanced disease. Pain can be a result of the tumor itself, metastasis, or cancer therapy, including chemotherapy and radiation therapy. Patients with cancer also may experience pain from conditions unrelated to their cancer, such as arthritis (Paice, 2004).
2. What medication(s) is the patient taking? Obtain drug history.
3. Obtain history, including (McCaffery & Pasero, 1999)
   a. Precipitating factors
   b. Character of pain
      i. What does your pain feel like?
      ii. What words would you use to describe your pain (e.g., burning, stabbing, aching)?
   c. Location of pain
      i. Where is your pain?
      ii. Is there more than one site?
   d. Onset and duration
      i. When did the pain start?
      ii. How often does it occur?
      iii. Has the intensity changed?
   e. Intensity
      i. On a scale of 0–10, with 0 being no pain and 10 being the worst pain you can imagine, how would you rate your pain?
      ii. Is the intensity consistent?
      iii. What is your pain rating at its worse? What is your pain rating at its best?
   f. Aggravating and relieving factors
      i. What makes your pain worse?
      ii. What makes your pain better?
   g. Previous treatments
      i. What types of treatments have you tried to relieve your pain?

      ii. Did these treatments help?

    h. Any associated symptoms, such as fever, swelling, or redness.

4. Past medical history
5. Changes in activities of daily living (i.e., Does the pain affect your physical and social function?)

Signs and Symptoms	Action
• Describe signs/symptoms of acute injury, spinal cord compression, pathological fracture, or other life-threatening problem. • Sudden onset of severe weakness or unrelenting localized pain; inability to ambulate, decreased sensation in extremities; loss of control of bowel or bladder (Wilkes, 2004) • Chest pain	Seek emergency care. Call ambulance immediately.
• Sudden onset of moderate to severe pain • Pain not responsive to current medication regimen • Pain that interferes with mobility	Seek medical care within two to four hours.
• Mild to moderate pain that has been increasing • Pain that is not controlled by current regimen • Pain that is interfering with activity or sleep	Seek urgent care within 24 hours.
• Mild aches and pains	Follow homecare instructions. Notify MD if no improvement.

HOMECARE INSTRUCTIONS

- Take acetaminophen, aspirin, or ibuprofen per label instructions for mild pain as recommended by physician (American Pain Society, 2003).
- Take prescription analgesics as prescribed.
- Maintain activity as tolerated.
- Keep pain diary, including description of the pain, character, severity, location; interventions taken; nonpharmacologic and pain medication taken; evaluation of response to interventions.
- Nonpharmacologic interventions (McCaffery & Pasero, 1999)
  - Heat or cold
  - Distraction therapy using music, hobbies. This should be individualized to the patient.

- Visualization
- Guided imagery
- Massage

Report the Following Problems

- No improvement in pain
- Pain that does not subside with interventions
- Other side effects, such as sedation, nausea, and constipation

Seek Emergency Care Immediately if Either of the Following Occurs

- Excruciating pain
- Immobility

REFERENCES

American Pain Society. (2003). *Principles of analgesic use in the treatment of acute pain and chronic cancer pain* (5th ed.). Skokie, IL: Author.

McCaffery, M., & Pasero, C. (1999). *Pain: Clinical manual.* St. Louis, MO: Mosby.

Paice, J.A. (2004). Pain. In C.H. Yarbro, M.H. Frogge, & M. Goodman (Eds.), *Cancer symptom management* (3rd ed., pp. 77–96). Sudbury, MA: Jones and Bartlett.

Thomas, C.L. (Ed.) (1997). *Taber's cyclopedic medical dictionary* (18th ed.). Philadelphia: F.A. Davis.

Wilkes, G.M. (2004). Spinal cord compression. In C.H. Yarbro, M.H. Frogge, & M. Goodman (Eds.), *Cancer symptom management* (3rd ed., pp. 359–374). Sudbury, MA: Jones and Bartlett.

Melanie Simpson, RN, BSN, OCN®, CHPN
Nurse Clinician, Pain Management Resource Team
University of Kansas Hospital
Kansas City, KS

Paresthesia (peripheral neuropathy)

PROBLEM

Paresthesia is characterized by numbness and tingling and is a common symptom of peripheral neuropathy. Peripheral neuropathy is a disturbance in the peripheral nervous system that results in sensory, motor, autonomic, or cranial nerve dysfunction. Associated symptoms include dysesthetic pain, loss of temperature sensation, loss of position sense, loss of vibratory sense, weakness, and ataxia (Boyle, 2000; Wilkes, 2004).

ASSESSMENT CRITERIA

(Boyle, 2000; Nielsen & Brant, 2002; Sweeney, 2002; Wilkes, 2004)

1. What is the cancer diagnosis and treatment?
   Peripheral neuropathy may result from direct damage from neurotoxic chemotherapy agents, including vinca alkaloids, heavy metals (e.g., cisplatin), and taxanes. Indirect damage can occur from compression of a nerve associated with metastasis or compression fracture. Other risk factors include age (> 60 years old), concurrent use of neurotoxic drugs, radiation therapy to spinal fields, diabetes mellitus, malnutrition with vitamin deficiency (B complex), and alcohol abuse.
2. What medication(s) is the patient taking? Obtain drug history.
3. Ask patient to describe symptoms in detail.
   a. Sensation(s)
   b. Any associated symptoms
4. Obtain history, including
   a. Precipitating factors
   b. Onset and duration
      Symptoms occurring for years suggest hereditary cause, occurring from weeks to months suggest drug-related toxicity or metabolic cause, occurring for days suggest chemotherapy toxicity or Guillain-Barré syndrome.
   c. Relieving factors
   d. Any associated symptoms, such as inability to move, pain, constipation, abdominal distress, incontinence, urinary retention.
5. Past medical history
   a. Diabetes mellitus
   b. Malnutrition
   c. Alcohol abuse

6. Changes in activities of daily living, such as difficulty handling keys, tying shoes, buttoning shirt, or tripping

Signs and Symptoms	Action
• Complete loss of feeling and movement • Pain with and without movement • Bedridden	Seek emergency care. Call ambulance immediately.
• Paresthesia interfering with activities of daily living • Pain with activities • Unable to distinguish temperature sensations • Unilateral paresthesia	Seek urgent care within 24 hours.
• Paresthesia including tingling, loss of deep tendon reflexes but interfering with < 25% of function and not interfering with activities of daily living (Sweeney, 2002)	Follow homecare instructions. Notify MD if no improvement

Cross references: Constipation, Difficulty or Pain With Urination, Pain

HOMECARE INSTRUCTIONS

(Boyle, 2000; Sweeney, 2002; Wilkes, 2004)

- Wear socks and shoes to protect feet.
- Apply non-skid surfaces on floors and tubs.
- Continue walking or other mild exercise.
- Use a potholder or oven mitts when cooking.
- Use gloves when washing dishes or gardening.
- Inspect skin for cuts, abrasions, and burns daily.
- Keep rooms well lit.
- Use handrails on stairs.
- Use a thermometer to check temperature of bath water. Avoid extreme temperatures.
- Use caution when driving and operating machinery.
- Vitamin B_6 may improve symptoms if prescribed by physician.

Report the Following Problem

- Worsening of numbness, tingling, pain, or loss of function

Seek Emergency Care Immediately if Any of the Following Occurs

- Burns
- Uncontrolled bleeding from injuries

- Infection of wounds
- Unrelieved pain
- Sudden loss of function or sensation

REFERENCES

Boyle, D.M. (2000). Peripheral neuropathy. In D. Camp-Sorrell & R.A. Hawkins (Eds.), *Clinical manual for the oncology advanced practice nurse* (pp. 751–757). Pittsburgh, PA: Oncology Nursing Society.

Nielsen, E., & Brant, J. (2002). Chemotherapy-induced neurotoxicity. *American Journal of Nursing, 102*(Suppl. 4), 16–19.

Sweeney, C.W. (2002). Understanding peripheral neuropathy in patients with cancer: Background and patient assessment. *Clinical Journal of Oncology Nursing, 6,* 163–166.

Wilkes, G. (2004). Peripheral neuropathy. In C.H. Yarbro, M.H. Frogge, & M. Goodman (Eds.), *Cancer symptom management* (3rd ed., pp. 333–358). Sudbury, MA: Jones and Bartlett.

Patricia I. Geddie, RN, MS, AOCN®
Education Coordinator II/Specialist
M.D. Anderson Cancer Center Orlando
Orlando, FL

Phlebitis

PROBLEM

Inflammation of a vein

ASSESSMENT CRITERIA

1. What is the cancer diagnosis and treatment?
   Is patient currently being treated with IV therapy that can irritate a vein causing phlebitis (Camp-Sorrell, 2000)?
2. What medication(s) is the patient taking? Obtain drug history.
3. Recent history of IV therapy
4. Ask patient to describe symptoms in detail.
   a. Discomfort
   b. Location of problem—old IV site, central line site
   c. Appearance of the area
      Common appearance of hard cord-like area along the vein; warmth, redness, tenderness, and swelling along vein, drainage
   d. Appearance of the site and limb
5. Obtain history, including
   a. Precipitating factors
   b. Onset and duration
   c. Relieving factors
   d. Any associated symptoms such as redness, swelling, ulceration, drainage, or fever.
6. Past medical history
   a. History of phlebitis
   b. Recent dehydration (Dehydration may contribute because of increase in blood viscosity.)
7. Changes in activities of daily living

Signs and Symptoms	Action
• Sudden chest pain or shortness of breath	Seek emergency care. Call ambulance immediately.
• Ulceration or purulent drainage from site • Red streak migrating from area of concern	Seek urgent care within 24 hours.

(Continued on next page)

(Continued)

Signs and Symptoms	Action
• Limb is swollen outside of area of concern. • Presence of fever	Seek urgent care within 24 hours.
• Redness, tenderness, and swelling at an IV site (current or in the past)	Follow homecare instructions. Notify MD if no improvement.

Cross references: Deep Venous Thrombosis, Dyspnea, Fever
Note. Based on information from Camp-Sorrell, 2000.

HOMECARE INSTRUCTIONS

(Camp-Sorrell, 2000)

• Treat with warm soaks for 20 minutes at a time four times a day.
• Elevate affected area for 72 hours.
• Perform gentle arm exercises (if site is in the arm or hand).
• For pain, take nonsteroidal anti-inflammatory drugs, as prescribed by physician.

Report the Following Problems

• A red streak develops moving upward from site.
• Ulcer or wound develops at site.
• Limb becomes swollen.
• Symptoms worsen.
• No relief is seen within 48–72 hours.
• Fever develops.

Seek Emergency Care Immediately if Either of the Following Occurs

• Sudden chest pain
• Shortness of breath

REFERENCE

Camp-Sorrell, D. (2000). Phlebitis. In D. Camp-Sorrell & R.A. Hawkins (Eds.), *Clinical manual for the oncology advanced practice nurse* (pp. 945–946). Pittsburgh, PA: Oncology Nursing Society.

Margaret Hickey, RN, MSN, MS, OCN®, CORLN

Pruritus (itch)

PROBLEM

Excessive itching of the skin

ASSESSMENT CRITERIA

(Fleischer & Dalgleish, 2002; Lester, 2000; Physician Data Query, 2003)

1. What is the cancer diagnosis and treatment?
   Pruritus is more common in the following cancers: hematologic malignancies, Hodgkin's disease, lymphoma, sarcomas, and visceral tumors.
2. What medication(s) is the patient taking? Obtain drug history.
   Consider allergic reaction, opioids, antibiotics, and contraceptives.
3. Ask patient to describe symptoms in detail.
4. Obtain history, including
   a. Precipitating factors
   b. Onset and duration
   c. Relieving factors
   d. Any associated symptoms.
5. Past medical history
   a. Liver disease
   b. Infection
6. Changes in activities of daily living and levels of stress

Signs and Symptoms	Action
• Difficulty breathing • Chest tightness or pain • Sense of overwhelming anxiety or "impending doom"	Seek emergency care. Call ambulance immediately.
• Generalized rash with wheals or hives or without generalized itching • Fever • Pustules or lesions with exudate • Pustules along a nerve track • Bleeding • Jaundice	Seek urgent care within two hours.

(Continued on next page)

(Continued)

Signs and Symptoms	Action
• Pain • Introduction of a new medication or complementary therapy within the past 24 hours	Seek urgent care within two hours.
• Localized rash with or without localized itching • Scaling • Cracking • Scratch marks or breaks in skin • Inflammation • Scabies or lice • White or red patches on skin • Exposure to a new animal, plant, or chemical within the past two days.	Seek urgent care within 24 hours.
• Itching without other symptoms	Follow homecare instructions. Notify MD if no improvement.

Cross reference: Rash
Note. Based on information from Fleischer & Dalgleish, 2002; Lester, 2000.

HOMECARE INSTRUCTIONS

(Fleischer & Dalgleish, 2002; Lester, 2000; Physician Data Query, 2003)

- Increase fluid intake.
- Use mild soaps or soaps made for sensitive skin.
- Oatmeal baths or soap may provide relief.
- Avoid perfumed soaps or bubble baths.
- Bathe only once a day in cool water.
- Apply skin emollients or lotions immediately after bathing while skin is still damp and then one or two times throughout the day.
- Avoid lotions containing alcohol. Lotions and emollients recommended for sensitive skin include Eucerin®, Alpha Keri®, Lubriderm® or Nivea®.
- Avoid tight, irritating clothing. Wear loose, soft cotton garments.
- Use mild laundry detergents, such as those designed for infants, when washing clothing and bed linens.

Report the Following Problems (Lester, 2000)

- Itchiness that continues for more than 48 hours after the above measures have been implemented
- Development of a rash, scaling, cracking, bleeding, redness, white patches, or blisters
- Temperature > 100.4°F

Seek Emergency Care Immediately if Any of the Following Occurs

- Chest tightness
- Difficulty breathing
- Generalized body rash with wheals or hives

REFERENCES

Fleischer, A., & Dalgleish, D. (2002). Pruritus. In A. Berger, R. Portenoy, & D. Weissman (Eds.), *Principles and practice of palliative care and supportive oncology* (2nd ed., pp. 299–306). Philadelphia: Lippincott Williams & Wilkins.

Lester, J. (2000). Pruritus. In D. Camp-Sorrell & R.A. Hawkins (Eds.), *Clinical manual for the oncology advanced practice nurse* (pp. 79–82). Pittsburgh, PA: Oncology Nursing Society.

Physician Data Query. (2003). *Supportive care: Pruritus.* Retrieved July 12, 2003, from http://www.cancer.gov

Jennifer S. Webster, MN, MPH, RN
Clinical Nurse Specialist/Nurse Practitioner
Georgia Cancer Specialists
Atlanta, GA

Rash

PROBLEM

An eruption of the skin (Murphy-Ende, 2000)

ASSESSMENT CRITERIA

1. What is the cancer diagnosis and treatment?
   A rash can result from a number of factors in a patient with cancer, including
   a. Drug induced from chemotherapy agents, including doxorubicin, mechlorethamine, cytarabine, bleomycin, cyclophosphamide, chlorambucil, methotrexate, melphalan, thiotepa, asparaginase, aldesleukin, interferon, 5-fluorouracil, capecitabine, antibiotics, epidermal growth factor receptors (Skidmore-Roth, 2004)
   b. Treatment related—radiation therapy skin changes
   c. Infectious—candidiasis, cellulitis, chicken pox, erythema multiforme, herpes simplex, herpes zoster, impetigo, measles, rubella, scabies, Lyme disease
   d. Allergic—atopic dermatitis, angioneurotic edema, contact dermatitis, drug allergies (see drug induced)
   e. Environmental—sunburn, chemical irritants, over washing/drying of skin, plant/animal exposure
   f. Autoimmune—cutaneous lupus, erythema nodosum, dermatomyositis, systemic lupus erythematosis, thrombocytopenic purpura
   g. Malignancy associated—abdominal/gastrointestinal, adrenocorticotropic hormone- (ACTH-) producing tumors, basal cell and squamous cell carcinoma, carcinoid, colon cancer, cutaneous T cell lymphoma, Kaposi's sarcoma, leukemia, melanoma, neurofibroma (Carucci & Leffell, 2002)
   h. Psychiatric—stress, anxiety, tension.
2. What medication(s) is the patient taking? Obtain drug and allergy history.
3. Ask patient to describe symptoms in detail.
   a. Onset of rash
   b. Location where rash first started
   c. Areas where rash spread
   d. Conjunctival involvement
   e. Color
   f. Texture: raised, flat, or blistered

    g. Change in character of rash with time

    h. Associated symptoms, such as itching, burning, numbness, or pain

    i. Aggravating factors, such as sunlight

    j. Alleviating factors and treatments tried

    k. Other associated symptoms, including fever, headache, malaise, arthralgia, conjunctivitis

    l. Contact with those who have a similar rash

    m. Recent travel

    n. Insect bites or stings

    o. New skin products used, such as lotion, soap, laundry detergent

    p. New medications

    q. Radiation therapy

    r. Pruritus

    s. Crusting of skin

    t. Pain, redness, warmth, tingling

    u. Drainage or "weeping"

4. Obtain history, including

    a. Precipitating factors

    b. Onset and duration

    c. Relieving factors

    d. Any associated symptoms, such as allergic reactions, infections, or systemic conditions.

5. Past medical history

    a. Exposure to people with a similar rash

    b. Diabetes

    c. Kidney disease

    d. Skin diseases, such as psoriasis

6. Changes in activities of daily living

Signs and Symptoms	Action
• Acute skin changes and associated systemic symptoms such as swelling of throat, stridor, wheezing, dyspnea, chest pain, severe headache, eye involvement, desquamation, high fever, mottled skin below the waist	Seek emergency care. Call ambulance immediately (Levinson, 2001).
• Dermatomal pain, itching, burning, paresthesia or hyperesthesia, rash over cranial nerves (herpes zoster pattern) • Stevens-Johnson syndrome: sudden eruption of erythematous macules, papules, vesicles, or bullae	Seek urgent care within 24 hours.

(Continued on next page)

(Continued)

Signs and Symptoms	Action
• Infection: drainage from lesion • Uncontrolled pruritus • History of new drug (suspected drug-induced rash) • Systemic symptoms associated with infections or viral syndrome, such as fever, myalgias, arthralgias	Seek urgent care within 24 hours.

• Chemotherapy-related signs or symptoms of hand-foot syndrome
  - See Hand-Foot Syndrome
  - Mild pruritus
  - Mild pain
• Low-grade fever and nonprogressive symptoms
	Follow homecare instructions. Notify MD if no improvement.

Cross references: Hand-Foot Syndrome, Pain, Pruritus	

HOMECARE INSTRUCTIONS

- Report changes in itching or rash to nurse.
- Report presence of drainage from skin lesions.
- Apply cool compresses to area.
- Apply topical medication as prescribed.
- Take oral medication as prescribed, and notify nurse of side effects; expect drowsiness from antihistamines, and take safety precautions.
- Wear loose-fitting cotton clothing.
- Keep fingernails cut short, and wear soft mittens at night to avoid scratching.
- Avoid hot baths and showers.
- Avoid sunlight and sunscreen protection.
- Hand-foot syndrome: Avoid hot water; elevate arms and feet; avoid rubbing and prolonged pressure to elbows, knees, hands, and feet; avoid tight-fitting shoes; avoid activities that place stress on hands and feet (Armstrong, Rust, & Kohtz, 1997) (see Hand-Foot Syndrome).
- Acute radiation therapy skin changes: Topical application of prescribed medication, application of dressing (hydrogel, hydrocolloid, or polyurethane film), cleansing of area with wound cleanser as prescribed by physician (Blackmar, 1997)

Report the Following Problems

- Rash progresses
- No improvement over the next three days

- Fever that persists for 24 hours
- Increasing pain or uncontrolled pruritus

Seek Emergency Care Immediately if Any of the Following Occurs
(Howard & White, 2001)

- Severe headache
- Difficulty breathing
- Chest pain
- High fever
- Eye involvement

REFERENCES

Armstrong, T., Rust, D., & Kohtz, J.R. (1997). Neurologic, pulmonary, and cutaneous toxicities of high-dose chemotherapy. *Oncology Nursing Forum, 24*(Suppl. 1), 23–33.

Blackmar, A. (1997). A focus on wound care: Radiation-induced skin alterations. *Medical/Surgical Nursing, 6*(3), 172–175.

Carucci, J., & Leffell, D. (2002). Treatment of tumor-related skin disorders. In A. Berger, R. Portenoy, & D. Weissman (Eds.), *Principles and practice of palliative care and supportive oncology* (pp. 307–320). Philadelphia: Lippincott Williams & Wilkins.

Howard, A., & White, C. (2001). Herpes labialis and herpes genitalis. In R. Rakel & E. Bope (Eds.), *Conn's current therapy* (pp. 846–850). Philadelphia: Saunders.

Levinson, A. (2001). Anaphylaxis and serum sickness. In R. Rakel & E. Bope (Eds.), *Conn's current therapy* (pp. 773–776). Philadelphia: Saunders.

Murphy-Ende, K. (2000). Rash. In D. Camp-Sorrell & R.A. Hawkins (Eds.), *Clinical manual for the oncology advanced practice nurse* (pp. 83–90). Pittsburgh, PA: Oncology Nursing Society.

Skidmore-Roth, L. (2004). *Mosby's nursing drug reference*. St. Louis, MO: Mosby.

Kathleen Murphy-Ende, RN, PhD, AOCN®
Nurse Practitioner and Clinical Assistant Professor
University of Wisconsin Hospitals and Clinics
University of Wisconsin-Madison School of Nursing
Madison, WI

Seizures

PROBLEM

An abrupt alteration in neurologic function caused by excessive activation of neurons (Minchin, 2000). Seizures are characterized by sudden, episodic, violent, involuntary muscle contractions resulting from the excessive discharge of cerebral neurons (Minchin).

Seizures may be classified as (Greenburg, Aminoff, & Simon, 2002; Hickey, 2003)
1. Generalized
   a. Tonic-clonic (grand mal)
   b. Absence (petit mal)
2. Partial
   a. Simple partial seizures
   b. Complex partial seizures
   c. Partial seizures with secondary generalization.

ASSESSMENT CRITERIA

1. What is the cancer diagnosis and treatment?
   Does the patient have a brain tumor or a cancer that commonly metastasizes to the brain? Common causes of seizure in patients with cancer include mass lesions (primary brain tumor, metastasis), central nervous system (CNS) hemorrhage, carcinomatous/lymphomatous meningitis, CNS infection (bacterial, viral, fungal, parasitic), encephalitis, hepatic encephalopathy, hypoxemia, metabolic abnormalities (hypoglycemia, hypomagnesemia, hyponatremia, hypernatremia, hyperosmolar states, hypocalcemia, uremia), or drug overdose (Glantz & Edwards, 2003; Parent & Aminoff, 2001; Waller & Caroline, 2000).
2. What medication(s) is the patient taking? Obtain drug history.
   a. Is the patient taking antiepileptic drugs? Have serum drug levels been monitored?
   b. Seizures may occur from toxic effects of drug therapy, such as from antidepressants, antipsychotics, insulin, cyclosporine, tacrolimus, etoposide, ifosfamide, cisplatinum, imipenem, or levofloxacin (Armstrong, Kanusky & Gilbert, 2003; Greenburg et al., 2002; Rosenfeld & Dalmau, 2002).
3. Review past medical history, including history of epilepsy, mental retardation, head trauma, HIV, or history of recent infection (Minchin, 2000; Parent & Aminoff, 2001).

4. Ask patient or significant other to describe symptoms in detail. Evaluate if the following occurred: Aura or change in consciousness prior to the event; an unusual feeling or smell prior to the seizure, a postictal state characterized by somnolence, confusion, or headache following the seizure; or amnesia following the event (Greenburg et al., 2002).

5. Obtain history of symptoms, including
   a. Severity—When did the seizure begin? How did it proceed?
   b. Precipitating factors.
      Seizures may be provoked by states that reduce the seizure threshold, such as fever, fatigue, stress, alcohol intake, and certain medications (Rosenfeld & Dalmau, 2002).
   c. Onset and duration—Was the onset abrupt? How long did the seizure last?
   d. Relieving factors
   e. Any associated symptoms—changes in muscle tone, posture, and muscle movement, aura prior to seizure activity, postictal somnolence.

6. Changes in activities of daily living

Signs and Symptoms	Action
• Sudden grand mal seizure activity, with or without loss of consciousness, loss of bowel or bladder control, and confusion • Seizure unrelieved by usual measures • Seizures accompanied by fever, bleeding, or new neurologic symptoms, such as headache, visual changes, or focal weakness • If patient sustained any injury as a result of the seizure	Seek emergency care. Call ambulance immediately.
• Known seizure disorder and experiences a typical event with recovery • Signs to suggest other clinical conditions that may have provoked the seizure, such as fever, intracranial hemorrhage, and fluid and electrolyte disturbance • New neurologic symptoms, such as headache, visual changes, focal weakness, sensory changes, or cognitive disturbance that suggest recurrence or progression of tumor	Seek care within 24 hours.
• Simple partial seizure: focal neurologic event with no impairment of consciousness	Seek care within 24–48 hours.

(Continued on next page)

(Continued)

Signs and Symptoms	Action
• Absence seizures (formerly called petit mal) that are brief and have no obvious motor symptoms	Seek care within 24–48 hours.

Cross reference: Confusion (change in level of consciousness)
Note. Based on information from Frucht & Bleck, 2002; Glantz & Edwards, 2003; Greenburg et al., 2002; Hickey, 2003; Parent & Aminoff, 2001; Waller & Caroline, 2000.

HOMECARE INSTRUCTIONS

- Avoid alcohol while taking anticonvulsants (Armstrong et al., 2003; Hickey, 2003).
- Seizure medications may be teratogenic; practice birth control (Greenburg et al., 2002).
- Antiepileptic drugs should not be discontinued abruptly because seizure frequency may increase. If anticonvulsants are to be withdrawn, each drug is tapered over two to four weeks (Minchin, 2000).
- Do not drive a car or operate complex machinery until patient gains sufficient experience with the effects of an antiepileptic drug to gauge whether it affects his or her mental and/or motor performance adversely.
- State laws vary regarding driving restrictions for patients who have had seizures (Krauss, Ampaw, & Krumholz, 2001).
  - Some states require healthcare providers to report patients with seizures to the division of motor vehicles.
  - Some states require a seizure-free period of varying length before the patient can drive again.
- Referral to an epilepsy center may be helpful for patients who have persistent seizures despite use of anticonvulsant medications (Minchin, 2000).
- Patients on an antiepileptic drug should have complete blood count and serum chemistries, including liver enzymes, which should be obtained at regular intervals to monitor for hematopoietic, renal, or hepatic dysfunction (Flowers, 2002).
- Antiepileptic drug levels should be monitored at intervals and whenever the patient reports symptoms that may suggest subtherapeutic or supratherapeutic blood levels (Glantz & Edwards, 2003; Natsch et al., 1997; Riva, Albani, Contin, & Baruzzi, 1996).

Seek Emergency Care Immediately if Any of the Following Occurs

- Tonic-clonic seizure activity lasting longer than five minutes; multiple seizures occurring without recovery and consciousness does not return; or complex partial seizure lasting longer than 30 minutes (Frucht & Bleck, 2002)
- Bruising

- Bleeding
- Rash
- Abdominal pain
- Vomiting
- Jaundice
- Lethargy
- Coma
- Marked increase in seizure frequency

REFERENCES

Armstrong, T.S., Kanusky, J.T., & Gilbert, M.R. (2003). Seize the moment to learn about epilepsy in people with cancer. *Clinical Journal of Oncology Nursing, 7,* 163–169.

Flowers, A. (2002). Seizures and syncope in the cancer patient. In V. Levin (Ed.), *Cancer in the nervous system* (2nd ed., pp. 438–453). New York: Oxford University Press.

Frucht, M., & Bleck, T. (2002). Seizures in the ICU patient. In N. Delanty (Ed.), *Seizures: Medical causes and management* (pp. 309–318). Totowa, NJ: Humana Press.

Glantz, M., & Edwards, K. (2003). The epidemiology and management of seizures in patients with cancer. In D. Schiff & P. Wen (Eds.), *Cancer neurology in clinical practice* (pp. 9–16). Totowa, NJ: Humana Press.

Greenburg, D.A., Aminoff, M.J., & Simon, R.P. (2002). *Clinical neurology* (5th ed.). New York: Lange Medical Books/McGraw-Hill.

Hickey, J. (2003). Seizures and epilepsy. In J. Hickey (Ed.), *The clinical practice of neurological and neurosurgical nursing* (5th ed., pp. 619–640). Philadelphia: Lippincott Williams & Wilkins.

Krauss, G.L., Ampaw, L., & Krumholz, A. (2001). Individual state driving restrictions for people with epilepsy in the U.S. *Neurology, 57,* 1780–1785.

Minchin, A.C. (2000). Seizures. In D. Camp-Sorrell & R.A. Hawkins (Eds.), *Clinical manual for the oncology advanced practice nurse* (pp. 805–810). Pittsburgh, PA: Oncology Nursing Society.

Natsch, S., Hekster, Y.A., Keyser, A., Decker, C.L., Meinardi, H., & Renier, W.O. (1997). Newer anticonvulsant drugs: Role of pharmacology, drug interactions and adverse reactions in drug choice. *Drug Safety, 17,* 228–240.

Parent, J.M., & Aminoff, M.J. (2001). Seizures and general medical disorders. In M. Aminoff (Ed.), *Neurology and general medicine* (3rd ed., pp. 967–981). New York: Churchill Livingstone.

Riva, R., Albani, F., Contin, M., & Baruzzi, A. (1996). Pharmacokinetic interactions between antiepileptic drugs: Clinical considerations. *Clinical Pharmacokinetics, 31,* 470–493.

Rosenfeld, M., & Dalmau, J. (2002). Seizures in cancer patients. In N. Delanty (Ed.), *Seizures: Medical causes and management* (pp. 207–232). Totowa, NJ: Humana Press.

Waller, A., & Caroline, N. (2000). *Handbook of palliative care in cancer* (2nd ed.). Philadelphia: Butterworth-Heinemann Medical.

Sandra A. Mitchell, CRNP, MScN, AOCN®
Oncology Nurse Practitioner
National Cancer Institute
Bethesda, MD
Faculty Associate, School of Nursing
University of Maryland
Baltimore, MD

Taste Alterations

PROBLEM

Change of taste of foods

ASSESSMENT CRITERIA

(DeConno, Ripamonti, Sbanotto, & Ventafridda, 1989; Grant & Kravits, 2000; Wickham et al., 1999)

1. What is the cancer diagnosis and treatment?
   Taste changes can result from surgical changes, radiation therapy to the head and neck area, and chemotherapy. Commonly reported changes include a decreased threshold for bitter, beef, pork, chocolate, coffee, or tomato. An increased threshold for sweet usually will lead the patient to add sugar to food, whereas a decreased threshold may cause an aversion to sweet foods. Other taste changes include an increased need for salt, avoidance of sour foods, or a metallic or medicinal taste.
2. What medication(s) is the patient taking? Obtain drug history—prescribed and over-the-counter medication—including vitamin supplements.
3. Ask patient to describe symptoms in detail.
   a. Sweet or sour aversions
   b. What tastes are affected?
   c. Is diet intake affected?
4. Obtain history, including
   a. Precipitating factors
   b. Onset and duration
   c. Relieving factors
   d. Any associated symptoms, such as weight loss, xerostomia, poor food or fluid intake, stomatitis, pain, dental caries, difficulty chewing or swallowing.
5. Past medical history
   a. Dental care
   b. Diabetes mellitus
6. Changes in activities of daily living
7. Diet history of typical 24-hour day prior to cancer diagnosis/treatment and current diet history

Signs and Symptoms	Action
• Swollen or bleeding gums, inability to swallow, or severe oral pain	Seek emergency care.
• Stomatitis, glossitis (raw tongue), atrophic lingua (slick tongue), or weight loss	Seek urgent care within 24 hours.
• Patient reports food tasting like cardboard or metal; food tastes too salty, sweet, sour, or bitter.	Follow homecare instructions. Notify MD if no improvement.

Cross references: Mucositis, Pain, Xerostomia

HOMECARE INSTRUCTIONS

(Bender, 1999; Brodie, 1998; Grant & Kravits, 2000; Sherry, 2002; Strohl, 1984; Stubbs, 1989)

- Increase your fluid intake to two to three liters a day. Drink nonirritating liquids, such as apple juice, grape juice, and sports drinks. Keep your mouth moist by spraying with water, artificial saliva, or saline.
- Suck on sugar-free sour candies to stimulate saliva production.
- Eat small, frequent meals.
- Use plastic utensils if food tastes metallic.
- Eat in pleasant surroundings with family and friends.
- Eat sugar-free mints, chew sugar-free gum, or chew ice to mask the bitter or metallic taste.
- Substitute poultry, fish, eggs, peanut butter, beans, and dairy products for red meats.
- Marinate meats in sweet fruit juices, wines, salad dressing, barbeque sauce, or sweet and sour sauces.
- Flavor foods with herbs, spices, sugar, lemon, and tasty sauce.
- Chilled or frozen food typically is more acceptable to patients than warm food.
- Do not eat one to two hours before chemotherapy or radiation therapy and up to three hours after therapy.
- Brush your teeth before and after each meal.
- Avoid cigarette smoking.
- Control noxious odors in the environment.

Report the Following Problems (Grant & Kravits, 2000)

- Weight loss
- Stomatitis

Seek Emergency Care Immediately if Any of the Following Occurs

- Uncontrolled bleeding from mouth
- Inability to swallow
- Severe pain in mouth

REFERENCES

Bender, C. (1999). Taste alteration. In J. Yasko (Ed.), *Nursing management of symptoms associated with chemotherapy* (4th ed., pp. 55–63). Bala Cynwyd, PA: Meniscus Health Care Communications.

Brodie, K. (1998). Taste alterations. In F. Preston & R. Cunningham (Eds.), *Clinical guidelines for symptom management in oncology* (pp. 73–77). New York: Clinical Insight Press.

De Conno, F., Ripamonti, C., Sbanotto, A., & Ventafridda, V. (1989). Oral complications in patients with advanced cancer. *Journal of Palliative Care, 5*(1), 7–15.

Grant, M., & Kravits, K. (2000). Symptoms and their impact on nutrition. *Seminars in Oncology Nursing, 16,* 113–121.

Sherry, V. (2002). Taste alterations among patients with cancer. *Clinical Journal of Oncology Nursing, 6,* 73–77.

Strohl, R. (1984). Understanding taste changes. *Oncology Nursing Forum, 11*(3), 81–84.

Stubbs, L. (1989). Taste changes in cancer patients. *Nursing Times, 85*(3), 49–50.

Wickham, R.S., Rehwaldt, M., Kefer, C., Shotts, S., Abbas, K., Glynn-Tucker, E., et al. (1999). Taste changes experienced by patients receiving chemotherapy. *Oncology Nursing Forum, 26,* 697–706.

Victoria Wenhold Sherry, MSN, CRNP
Inpatient Oncology Nurse Practitioner
The Hospital of the University of Pennsylvania
Philadelphia, PA

Venous Access Device Problems

PROBLEM

A tunneled central venous catheter, peripherally inserted central catheter (PICC), or implanted port with a problem noted by the patient. See Appendix D for ambulatory pump troubleshooting guide.

ASSESSMENT CRITERIA

(Camp-Sorrell, 2004)

1. What is the cancer diagnosis and treatment?
   Patients frequently are sent home with central venous catheters, including tunneled catheters (single and multiple lumen), PICC lines, or an implanted port. Tunneled catheters or PICC lines may be clamped off, with routine flushing performed by the patient, homecare agency, or clinic, or the patient may be on home IV infusion.
2. What is the central line being used for?
3. What medication(s) is the patient taking? Obtain drug history.
4. Ask patient to describe symptoms in detail.
   a. Is the site swollen, red, or tender?
   b. Is there any streaking present or a red or discolored line on the skin, or along the path of the catheter?
   c. Is there leakage?
      i. From where?
      ii. Amount of leakage?
      iii. Color of leakage?
   d. Is blood present in tubing or leaking?
   e. Is there a break in the tubing?
   f. Is there a change in the ability to infuse fluids or flush?
   g. Is there an odd sensation or gurgling in neck; arm or shoulder pain; or vague back discomfort?
5. Obtain history, including
   a. Precipitating factors
   b. Onset and duration
   c. Relieving factors
   d. Any associated symptoms, such as shortness of breath, swelling, pain, and drainage.
6. Past medical history
   a. Any history of infection

    b. Suspected neutropenia or thrombocytopenia
    c. Current or recent infusion of a vesicant
7. Changes in activities of daily living

Signs and Symptoms	Action
• Line open to air and patient short of breath • Site painful and vesicant infusing • Line dislodged/fell out and site bleeding	Clamp line immediately or apply pressure to site if line fell out. Seek emergency care. Call ambulance immediately.
• Line broken or leaking • Face, neck, exit site swelling • Inability to flush or to infuse fluid • Line fell out/dislodged • Headache related to infusions • Redness, swelling, tenderness, or streaks at insertion site • Drainage from exit site • Strange gurgling sensation in the neck; arm or shoulder pain; or vague back discomfort	Clamp IV line and seek urgent care within 24 hours.
• No blood return when IV tubing is pinched • Blood backing up in tubing	Follow homecare instructions. Notify MD if no improvement.

Note. Based on information from Briggs, 2002; Camp-Sorrell, 2004.

HOMECARE INSTRUCTIONS

(Briggs, 2002; Camp-Sorrell, 2004)

• Ensure patient/family is aware of signs and symptoms to report, such as problems with IV flow, leakage from line or site, and signs and symptoms of infection (fever, redness, swelling, or drainage at site).
• Ensure patient or family (home care or clinic) is aware of schedule and responsibility for flushing the line and dressing changes as needed.
• Check tubing for kinks and clamps.
• Change positions of body or arm.
• Raise bag if not on a pump.
• Check pump to make sure it is functioning properly (see Appendix D on ambulatory pumps).
• If instructed in flushing, flush the line slowly. If it flushes easily, flush more forcibly with 10 cc of normal saline solution.
• If line is broken externally, clamp the tube above break and contact homecare nurse or come to office.

Report the Following Problems (Briggs, 2002)

- Problem persists after homecare measures taken
- Signs of infection
- Signs of infiltration
- Persistent discomfort

Seek Emergency Care Immediately if Any of the Following Occurs

- Line open to air and patient short of breath
- Site painful and vesicant infusing
- Line dislodged with bleeding

REFERENCES

Briggs, J.K. (2002). *Telephone triage protocols for nurses* (2nd ed.). Philadelphia: Lippincott Williams & Wilkins.

Camp-Sorrell, D. (Ed.). (2004). *Access device guidelines: Recommendations for nursing practice and education* (2nd ed.). Pittsburgh, PA: Oncology Nursing Society.

Margaret Hickey, RN, MSN, MS, OCN®, CORLN

Xerostomia (dry mouth)

PROBLEM

Xerostomia, or hyposalivation, is dryness of the mouth. It can be a frequent complaint among the elderly, individuals with systemic diseases such as diabetes, and patients undergoing radiation therapy for head and neck cancers or total body irradiation, and it is a side effect of multiple medications. A reduction in saliva enhances the growth of microorganisms in the oral cavity, increases the incidence of periodontal disease, and alters a patient's sensation of taste and swallowing, thus decreasing optimal nutritional status (Holmes, 1998). In the immunosuppressed patient, the oral mucosa is the most frequently documented source of infection (Strohl, 2000).

ASSESSMENT CRITERIA

(Madeya, 1996; Strohl, 2000)

1. What is the cancer diagnosis and treatment?
    Xerostomia can be a result of radiation therapy or direct extension of the tumor. It also can result from chemotherapy and other medications. As a side effect of radiation therapy for head and neck cancers, xerostomia is not only reported while the patient is under treatment but also can persist six months after therapy is completed or can even be permanent. Prior to initiating radiotherapy to the head and neck area or chemotherapy that induces oral cavity changes, a dental consult should be obtained. The goal of symptom management includes maintaining mucosal integrity and minimizing oral or systemic infection.
2. What medication(s) is the patient taking? Obtain drug history.
    Xerostomia is a side effect of antidepressants, antihistamines, diuretics, anticholinergics, and opioids, as well as others. Chemotherapeutic agents include 5-fluorouracil, doxorubicin, vincristine, vinblastine, methotrexate, and cytarabine.
3. Obtain past medical history.
    a. Systemic diseases, such as diabetes
    b. Nutritional status
    c. Oral hygiene regimen
    d. Previous oral/dental disease (candidiasis, herpes)
4. Ask patient to describe symptoms.
    a. Quality of saliva (thin and watery versus thick and ropey)
    b. Dryness and/or coating on the lips, mucosa, or tongue

    c. Degree of mucositis: erythema, ulceration, or hemorrhage of the gums or mucosa

    d. Burning or pain of the oral mucosa

    e. Sensitivity of teeth and gums

    f. Swallowing difficulty/pain with swallowing

5. Obtain history of xerostomia, including

    a. Precipitating factors (medications, hot foods, wearing dentures)

    b. Onset and duration

    c. Relieving factors (frequent mouth care, sips of water throughout the day, moistened foods, sugarless gum or candy)

    d. Use of salivary substitutes or salivary gland stimulants

    e. Ability to wear dentures and rate comfort with eating.

6. Assess for nutritional plan of care.

    Patients should receive a complete nutrition evaluation by a registered dietitian prior to the initiation of therapy. Recommendations include calorie and protein requirements, food consistency options, vitamin replacement, and the use of supplements. Assess labs for albumin, prealbumin, and transferrin. Recommendations may include enteral support, the gastrointestinal tract being the preferred method of support.

Signs and Symptoms	Action
• Temperature > 100.4°F or higher; chills with neutropenia	Seek emergency care. Generally, xerostomia is not an emergent condition.
• Oral assessment indicates increase in inflammation, presence of ulceration (white patches, confluent patches). • Dizziness, increased weakness or fatigue • Decreased urine output that is cloudy or dark • Increased difficulty swallowing	Seek medical care within 24 hours.
• Oral assessment indicates dry lips and mucous membranes with thick secretions • Difficulty swallowing	Follow homecare instructions. Notify MD if no improvement.
Cross reference: Mucositis	

HOMECARE INSTRUCTIONS

- Follow nutrition plan as developed by registered dietitian.
- Carry water bottle throughout the day.

- Keep sugarless hard candies or sugarless gum on hand.
- Perform oral cavity assessment daily.
- Perform oral care after each meal and at bedtime or as directed. Use soft-bristle toothbrush; floss using waxed dental floss if no pain and if platelets are adequate; use alcohol-free mouth rinse.
- Use oral care agents, saliva substitutes, and salivary stimulants as directed.
- Use analgesics, anesthetics, and antibiotics as directed.
- Do not smoke or use alcohol.
- Maintain regular dental visits as directed.

Report the Following Problems (Strohl, 2000)

- Oral assessment indicates increase in inflammation, presence of ulceration (white patches, confluent patches).
- Dizziness, increased weakness/fatigue
- Decreased urine output that is cloudy or dark
- Increased difficulty swallowing

Seek Emergency Care Immediately if Either of the Following Occurs

- Temperature > 100.4°F
- Chills with neutropenia

REFERENCES

Holmes, S. (1998). Xerostomia: Etiology and management in cancer patients. *Supportive Care in Cancer, 6,* 348–355.

Madeya, M.L. (1996). Oral complications from cancer therapy: Part 2—nursing implications for assessment and treatment. *Oncology Nursing Forum, 23,* 808–818.

Strohl, R.A. (2000). Stomatitis/xerostomia. In D. Camp-Sorrell & R.A. Hawkins (Eds.), *Clinical manual for the oncology advanced practice nurse* (pp. 63–66). Pittsburgh, PA: Oncology Nursing Society.

Jackie Matthews, RN, MS, AOCN®
Oncology Clinical Nurse Specialist
Miami Valley Hospital
Dayton, OH

Karen Feldmeyer, RD, LD
Registered Licensed Dietitian
Department of Radiation Oncology
Miami Valley Hospital
Dayton, OH

Appendices

Appendix A. Telephone Triage Nursing and Management Policy—Department: Nursing

I. Background

Telephone triage is the process of ensuring the safe and effective disposition of patient health problems by telephone. Telephone triage nursing practice at the Cancer Institute of New Jersey (CINJ) is based on a commitment to the delivery of quality, cost-effective, and safe oncology care. Telephone triage nursing practice requires policies and organizational structure that provide mechanisms to ensure accountability, establish communication and reporting, and monitor the quality of the nursing service provided. Telephone triage policies are concordant with the standards mandated by regulatory agencies, the Nurse Practice Act of the State of New Jersey, and the guidelines of the Oncology Nursing Society (ONS).

CINJ has a designated telephone triage line, the Nurse Helpline. The Nurse Helpline at CINJ is staffed by an experienced oncology registered nurse. The purpose of the Nurse Helpline is to provide care to patients and families through assessment of actual or potential health needs, health promotion, education, counseling, and decision support and coordination of care. The line is available to patients from 9 am–5 pm, Monday through Friday. Patients access the Nurse Helpline via the central CINJ telephone number. Patients are referred to the answering service after hours or have the option to leave a message. All messages left on the Nurse Helpline are returned no later than the next business day.

II. Purpose

The purpose of this policy is to outline the process and management of the Nurse Helpline at CINJ.

III. Policy

A written position description has been developed for the telephone triage position. This document is consistent with state laws and the Nurse Practice Act, accepted standards of nursing practice, organizational policies, mission, values, and the performance evaluation system. Employee records are maintained with evidence of competency.

    A. Telephone nursing involves skills that include competency in critical thinking, expert clinical skills, as well as assessment and evaluation skills. Orientation to the triage line will be provided through an organized preceptor program using materials such as the Nurse Helpline's standard operating procedures, as outlined in this policy, and the Nurse Helpline Competency Checklist, among other materials. Educational opportunities are provided to maintain skills and address issues identified during quality improvement activities. The requirements for nurses who perform telephone triage and management are as follows:

        1. RN licensure in the state of New Jersey

        2. Current certification as an Oncology Certified Nurse (OCN®) or Advanced Oncology Certified Nurse (AOCN®)

        3. Successful completion of orientation to the Treatment Area as well as helpline-specific orientation as evidenced by completion of the Nurse Helpline Competency Checklist

(Continued on next page)

Appendix A. Telephone Triage Nursing and Management Policy—Department: Nursing *(Continued)*

    4. Demonstrated effective uses in clinical judgment and problem-solving skills, as demonstrated by a successful probationary evaluation

    5. Demonstrated effectiveness in communication skills with patients and colleagues

    6. Annual staff competency is determined by telephone call scenarios as demonstrated by the treatment nurse manager or designee "listening in" to a randomized sample of calls (N = 5 patients) by the nurse.

B. The scope of telephone nursing practice at CINJ includes

    1. Acute or emergent problems, with clear disposition requirements (e.g., call 911, refer to emergency room)

    2. Change in patient condition where intervention is designated by algorithm. Memorial Sloan-Kettering Cancer Center's (2000) *Ambulatory Care Telephone Triage and Symptom Management Protocol Manual* (2nd ed.) is utilized to guide practice.

    3. Questions related to patients' treatment plan (e.g., treatment schedule, anticipated toxicities, select laboratory, radiology test results)

    4. Patient education

    5. Nursing or protocol-specific interventions prescribed for pain, symptom, and medication management; homecare needs; and the nursing plan of care

    6. Questions about medical equipment, which may be referred to home care, as appropriate

    7. Lab or diagnostic testing results, which are within normal limits, as requested by the patient

    8. Notification of patients and provision of education related to management of the following changes in status: neutropenia (ANC < 1,000), thrombocytopenia (platelets < 30,000), or anemia (hemoglobin < 8.0).

C. Process improvement activities will be monitored annually and as needed by the Treatment Area nurse manager for each triage nurse using the Telephone Triage Quality Improvement Survey (see Appendix C). The process improvement activity involves interviewing a random sample of 5% of patients with whom the triage nurse has had recent contact.

D. Staffing patterns ensure that sufficient numbers of qualified staff are available to manage the complexity of patient calls. This number is based upon benchmark data from the healthcare industry, as well as from internal process improvement monitoring.

E. The process of telephone triage involves a series of specific steps. These include

    1. Assessment and data collection

    2. Analysis and synthesis of information, identification, and prioritization of the problem

    3. Intervention, including directives for where and when treatment should take place

    4. Documentation of the encounter

    5. Evaluation and follow-up.

F. An algorithm or protocol guides the process of telephone triage for the specific patient problem. The algorithms utilized at CINJ are adopted from

(Continued on next page)

Appendix A. Telephone Triage Nursing and Management Policy—Department: Nursing *(Continued)*

Memorial Sloan-Kettering Cancer Center's (2000) *Ambulatory Care Telephone Triage and Symptom Management Protocol Manual* (2nd ed.). These algorithms or protocols for telephone intervention are regularly reviewed and revised by Memorial Sloan-Kettering Cancer Center. The Ambulatory Care Board at CINJ approves the algorithms for use.

G. A standard Telephone Triage Documentation Form (Appendix B) is utilized to document all patient encounters except for laboratory and diagnostic study result and medical record requests, which are maintained in a patient log located at the Nurse Helpline. Records of all documentation are stored and are retrievable according to the organization's medical record standard. The "Telephone Triage Form" becomes a part of the patient's permanent medical record.

H. The triage documentation form requires the signature of either an advanced practice nurse (APN) or the attending physician. To facilitate the timely signing of forms, the following process will be implemented:
  1. The triage nurse will sort the triage documentation forms daily by attending physician.
  2. The sorted documentation forms will be maintained in an accordion file located in the Medical Record Department.
  3. The APN or physician will be required to review and sign the forms within 24 hours for their respective patients.
  4. The forms then will be placed in the medical record filing bin located in Medical Records for timely filing into the patient medical record.

I. Nurses practicing on the Nurse Helpline recognize the dignity and worth of individuals; respect cultural, spiritual, and psychosocial differences; and apply ethical concepts. Written organizational policies and procedures related to patients' rights and confidentiality are in place and outline the necessity of patient confidentiality during the telephone encounter and documentation of that encounter. The procedures include
  1. How to verify the identity of the person to whom the nurse is communicating over the phone.
      a) A password, distributed in the new patient information packet and verified at the patient's first visit, will be mandatory for providing patient-related information over the telephone.
      b) The password will be the patient's birth date.
      c) If the patient should forget the password, he or she will be asked to verify by utilizing his or her social security number.
      d) Provider or insurance company request for information must be submitted in writing on company letterhead.
  2. Appropriate use of answering machine/voice mail and faxing
      a) CINJ's general consent for care will contain a statement that permits CINJ to leave messages with an identified individual and/or on an answering machine. The patient will have the opportunity on the consent to designate the individual and a second phone number where he or she can be reached.
      b) If for some reason, by omission, the patient did not complete that section of the consent, the following situations would warrant the need for the triage nurse to leave a message with a significant

(Continued on next page)

Appendix A. Telephone Triage Nursing and Management Policy—Department: Nursing *(Continued)*

other and/or on an answering machine regardless of having written patient consent:

    (1)   Neutropenia

    (2)   Anemia

    (3)   Other abnormal laboratory values that could pose a risk to the patient (e.g., abnormal chemistry results)

    (4)   Labs required to complete an ordered CT scan.

  c)   The triage nurse is responsible for faxing the following documents, according to CINJ operating policy and procedure:

    (1)   BUN and creatinine results to radiology groups for the scheduling of CAT scans

    (2)   Authorized prescriptions to appropriate pharmacies

    (3)   Authorizations to homecare agencies for care

    (4)   Prescription for procedures.

  d)   All other fax requests will rest with the appropriate department.

  e)   Disability claim forms will be completed and faxed by the appropriate APN/nurse coordinator.

3. Communication with minors

  a)   No message will be left with a minor—defined as a child less than 18 years of age.

  b)   The triage nurse will continue to call the patient back until the patient or designated other is available. Documentation in the medical record will reflect this.

4. Reporting recognized child, geriatric, or spousal abuse situations

  a)   If an abusive situation is suspected in the home or revealed to the triage nurse by the patient or family member, the nurse should follow University of Medicine and Dentistry of New Jersey (UMDNJ) policy on Suspected Abuse Reporting.

5. Reporting or calling 911 in potential suicide or violent situations

For potential suicidal situations

  a)   The triage nurse will attempt to keep the patient or caller on the telephone by instructing him or her not to hang up.

  b)   The triage nurse will elicit the support from another staff member to contact 911 on a separate telephone.

  c)   If the triage nurse is unable to identify the location of the call, 911 will trace the call.

  d)   The triage nurse will engage the caller in conversation until emergency medical assistance arrives.

  e)   Document per CINJ policy.

For violent situations

  a)   Assess if the caller has a safe place (e.g., locked room, closet) where he or she can go with the telephone. Obtain the location, and instruct him or her to wait there.

  b)   Follow the steps as listed above under "suicidal situations."

6. Using language relay services if needed

  a)   Assess CINJ Translator List for availability of staff to translate.

  b)   If translator is unavailable, utilize University Medical Group (UMG) policy to obtain a translator.

(Continued on next page)

Appendix A. Telephone Triage Nursing and Management Policy—Department: Nursing *(Continued)*

7. Resolving problem calls with supervisory/collegial help
   For patient-related issues, the following chain of command should be followed:
   a) Appropriate APN or nurse coordinator (if applicable)
   b) Physician
   c) The assistant director of ambulatory services and/or the director of ambulatory services
   d) The chief of medical, surgical, gynecological, radiology, or pediatric oncology; the deputy director
   e) All other issues should be referred to the appropriate departmental manager.
8. Confidential storage of documentation:
   a) Completed triage documentation forms will be placed in the Medical Records filing bin to be filed in a timely fashion. Standard operating procedures regarding confidentiality will be maintained.
9. How to respond to abusive callers (e.g., yelling, screaming, cursing, threatening calls)
   a) Attempt to locate the real problem.
   b) Tell the caller he or she will be assisted if he or she can calmly explain the situation.
   c) If the abusive behavior persists, instruct the caller that the call will be terminated if the abuse does not stop.
   d) If the call is terminated, instruct the caller you are terminating the call and refer the situation to the attending physician and/or advanced practice nurse.
   e) Document per CINJ policy.
J. Triage nurses must confer with or refer the patient to the appropriate physician or nurse practitioner for determination of disposition in specific situations in compliance with the scope of nursing practice in New Jersey. Any medical order received in these situations, such as a verbal order, must be documented and co-signed by the responsible physician or nurse practitioner per CINJ operating policy. The following situations require notification to the appropriate physician or advanced practice nurse:
   1. Acute or emergent problems where notification of a physician or advanced practice nurse is designated in the algorithm or protocol, including unrelieved pain
   2. Potential need for change in the medical treatment plan (medication or procedures)
   3. Prescription re-fills
   4. Abnormal radiology results that demonstrate a change in the patient's condition and/or abnormal tumor marker tests must be given to the patient by the attending physician or APN.

References

Briggs, J. (1997). *Telephone triage protocols for nurses.* Philadelphia: Lippincott.
Cooley, M.E., Lin, E.M., & Hunter, S.W. (1994). The ambulatory oncology nurse's role. *Seminars in Oncology Nursing, 10,* 245–253.
Memorial Sloan-Kettering Cancer Center. (2000). *Ambulatory care telephone triage and symptom management protocol manual* (2nd ed.). New York: Author.

Note. Courtesy of the Cancer Institute of New Jersey. Used with permission.

Appendix B. Sample Telephone Triage Documentation Forms

UCLA Gynecology/Oncology Service   Date:
Chemotherapy Telephone Protocol   Time:

Patient: Doctor: Person receiving call:

Diagnosis	Phone number	Age
Chemo	Last course Total # treatments	Recent lab work
Recent illness/surgery		

Chief complaint

Onset	Location
Character	Duration
Associated factors	Receiving factors
Treatment tried	Current Meds

Emotional status:

Recommendations:

Pharmacy:

Allergies

Verbal contact/understanding   Follow-up:
with patient/family members:

Note. From "Outpatient Chemotherapy: Telephone Triage for Symptom Management," by P.J. Anastasia and M.C. Blevins, 1997, *Oncology Nursing Forum, 24*(Suppl. 1), p. 23. Copyright by the Oncology Nursing Society. Reprinted with Permission.

Appendix B. Sample Telephone Triage Documentation Forms

Telephone Triage Encounter Form

Date: _____ Time: _____   Caller: _____

Primary MD: _____   Agency: _____

❐ Triage to: _____   Patient: _____

Pharmacy name/number: _____   D.O.B. _____

❐ Returned call   Home: _____

❐ Will call again on: _____   Work: _____

                                   Pager/cell: _____

❐ Call results: Lab/date: _____ X-rays/date: _____ Path/date: _____

Dx: _____ ❐ TX   ❐ XRT   ❐ CRX   ❐ Other   FU: _____

Chief complaint: _____
_____
_____

Message Taken By: _____ ❐ **Chart Requested**

❐ **Emergent**   ❐ **Urgent**   ❐ **Non Urgent**

CVAD: _____ Allergy: _____ ❐ Med. Reviewed

Time call returned: _____
▶Onset ▶Location ▶Duration ▶Character ▶Associated factors ▶Relieving factors ▶Treatment tried

Data: _____
_____
_____

Action: _____
_____
_____

Response: _____
_____
_____

Patient/caregiver agrees to plan of care   ❐ Yes   ❐ No

RN _____ RN _____

(Continued on next page)

Appendix B. Sample Telephone Triage Documentation Forms

Telephone Triage Encounter Form (cont.)

Response: _____

_____

_____

_____

_____

_____

_____

_____

_____

_____

_____

_____

_____

_____

_____

_____

_____

_____

_____

_____

_____

_____

_____

_____

_____

_____

_____

Patient response: Patient/caregiver agrees to plan of care.　❑ Yes　　❑ No

RN: _____　RN: _____

Date: _____　Date: _____

```
Patient ID Label
```

Note. Courtesy of St. Luke's Mountain States Tumor Institute. Used with permission.

Appendix B. Sample Telephone Triage Documentation Forms

Telephone Triage Record

Date: ____ Time Received: _____ Time Completed: _____ ☐ Incoming ☐ Message

Patient Name: _____ Telephone Number: _____

Person Calling: _____ Relationship: _____

Physician: _____ Allergies: _____ Leave Message: ☐ Yes ☐ No

Chief Complaint: _____
_____
_____
_____
_____

Pain: ☐ Yes ☐ No   Location: _____ Intensity (0–10 scale): _____

Current Medications: _____

Action Taken: _____
_____
_____
_____
_____

Caller verbalizes understanding of instruction given: ☐ Yes ☐ No
Caller agrees with action taken: ☐ Yes ☐ No
Patient instructed to call if symptoms increase or change: ☐ Yes ☐ No
Does the caller require a call back? ☐ Yes ☐ No Call back date/time: _____

F/U call results/signature: _____
_____
_____ Date/Time _____

Pharmacist Name: _____ Telephone Number: _____
Pharmacy: _____ Address: _____
Drug: _____ Dose: _____
Frequency: _____ Dispense: _____ Refill: _____

Action Taken: Prescription: Called in ☐   Prescription Refilled ☐   Patient Notified ☐
Prescription Mailed ☐   Prescription Faxed ☐ _____

APN/MD notified: _____ Date/Time: _____
Triage Nurse Signature: _____ Date/Time: _____
APN/MD Signature: _____ Date/Time: _____

Note. Courtesy of the Cancer Institute of New Jersey. Used with permission.

Appendix B. Sample Telephone Triage Documentation Forms

Medical Oncology Hematology
Telephone Documentation

Date: _____

Message taken by: _____   Time: _____

Patient name: _____

Urgency
Emergency ☐
ASAP ☐
Today ☐

Reason for call
(patient's own words): _____
_____
_____
_____
_____

Problem: _____
_____
_____
_____
_____

Assessment: _____
_____
_____
_____
_____

Action taken: _____
_____
_____
_____
_____

Follow-up: _____

MD consulted: _____

Signature: _____

Note. Courtesy of Medical Oncology Hematology Associates, Inc. Used with permission.

Appendix C. Telephone Triage Quality Improvement Survey

Patient name: _____ Telephone #: _____

Date/time of initial call: _____ / _____

Question	Yes	No	Comments
Was the nurse courteous and professional?			
Were you comfortable with the advice given?			
Did you follow the advice given?			
Were you provided adequate referral information?			
Would you use the Nurse Helpline again?			

Comments: _____
_____
_____
_____
_____
_____
_____
_____

Follow-up: _____
_____
_____
_____
_____
_____
_____
_____
_____

_____   _____
Surveyor name   Date and time of call

Note. Courtesy of the Cancer Institute of New Jersey. Used with permission.

Appendix D. Sample of Patient Education Form for Patients Receiving Home Infusion Via Pump

PATIENT INSTRUCTIONS – AMBULATORY INFUSION

You have been provided with an AIM Plus infusion pump – serial # _____

Every day you must:
☐ Check that the small boxes are walking across your lower screen.
☐ Check that the numbers on the screen are counting up.
☐ Check that the bag volume is decreasing.

Troubleshooting:
☐ If "LOW BATTERIES" is displayed on the screen, press SILENCE, press STOP, replace batteries and follow screen instructions to "USE CURRENT THERAPY," press START to infuse. Verify that boxes are walking across the lower screen. Should you require any assistance with changing your batteries or if this is your first time, please call the InfuSystem Hotline at 1-800-962-9656, for clinician assistance.
☐ To quiet an alarm, press the SILENCE key and follow the prompts on the screen. If at any time you are unsure about correcting an alarm condition, just call 1-800-962-9656.
☐ When "ALMOST EMPTY" appears on the screen, delivery of your medicine will complete in 30 minutes or less. Do **NOT** stop the medicine. You may press SILENCE to mute the alarm for 10 minutes. When the pump has delivered the container amount programmed, the words "EMPTY CONTAINER" will appear on the screen. You will be scheduled to return to the office before this time.

Do's & Don'ts:
☐ Do check pump daily (more often if pump is programmed for less than 48 hours).
☐ When bathing, hang pump outside of shower. Do **not** submerge pump in water.
☐ Don't get dressing or pump wet.
☐ Don't drop the pump or strike against hard surfaces.
☐ Don't hesitate to call for pump troubleshooting assistance at 1-800-962-9656.
☐ Do read "Handling Chemotherapy Drugs Safely at Home," NIH publication regarding spills.

Port Care:
☐ If you notice that the area surrounding your port is red, swollen, draining or tender, please call the clinic at: .

Additional Instructions:
_____
_____

_____
Patient/Caregiver Signature   Date

_____
Nurse/Instructor Signature   Date

Important Phone Contact:
If you have a medical problem, please call our office:

If you have a pump problem, please call InfuSystem 24-hour support hotline at: 1-800-962-9656

Note. Courtesy of InfuSystem Ambulatory Infusion Devices. Used with permission.

Index

The letter *f* after a page number indicates that relevant content appears in a figure; the letter *t,* in a table.

A

AAACN. *See* American Academy of Ambulatory Care Nursing
AAON. *See* American Association of Office Nurses
abbreviations, avoidance of, 22
absence seizures, 189, 191
absolute neutrophil count (ANC), 125–126
abusive callers, 28
acetaminophen, 134, 165, 172
active listening, 27
ADA. *See* Americans with Disabilities Act
Addison's disease, 93
Agency for Healthcare Research and Quality (AHRQ), 21–22
AHRQ. *See* Agency for Healthcare Research and Quality
AIDS, 129
ALARM Model for Assessment of Sexual Functioning, 61
alcohol abuse, 175
aldesleukin, 185
algorithms, for telephone triage, 21
allergic reactions, 181, 185
alopecia, 57–59
alpha interferon, 141
Alpha Keri® lotion, 182
alprazolam, 68
ambulatory nursing, 1
ambulatory pump, 199, 218
American Academy of Ambulatory Care Nursing (AAACN), 7, 17, 38, 44, 46, 52
American Association of Office Nurses (AAON), 38, 46
American Cancer Society, 62, 95
American College of Emergency Physicians, 38
American Nursing Association (ANA), 7, 38
Americans with Disabilities Act (ADA), 38
amitriptyline, 150
ANA. *See* American Nursing Association

analgesics, 119, 121, 134, 165, 172
angioneurotic edema, 185
anorexia, 63–65
answering machines, 28, 33–34, 49
antacids, 97, 117, 119
antibiotics, 97, 117, 163, 181, 185
anticholinergics, 201
anticoagulants, 75–76, 90
anticonvulsants, 189, 191
antidepressants, 94, 201
  constipation from, 83
  seizures from, 189
antiemetics, 97
antihistamines, 68, 134, 201
antihypertensives, 97, 121
antipsychotics, 189
anxiety, 67–69, 114
anxiolytics, 67–68
appetite stimulants, 64
Arkansas State Board of Nursing, telenursing position statements of, 40–41
arthralgia, 134, 163–166
ascites, 71–73
asparaginase, 185
aspirin, 165, 172
assessment phase, of telephone triage, 12, 17–18, 33–35, 42, 51
assistive personnel (AP), 43
atrophic lingua, 194
autoimmune disorders, 185

B

baclofen, 150
Bag Balm® cream, 138
BCG treatment, for bladder cancer, 101–102, 145
benzodiazepines, 68
biological response modifiers (BRMs), 141
bladder cancer, hematuria with, 145
bleeding/blood, 75–77, 84, 99, 155, 193
  in emesis, 168
  in urine. *See* hematuria
bleomycin, 185
boards of nursing, 38–42
body image, 93

bradykinin, 163
breast lump/tenderness, 156
BRMs (biological response modifiers), 141
bruising, 75–76

C

calf, pain in, 90, 155
California State Board of Nursing, telenursing position statements of, 41
callbacks, 26, 31–32, 35, 47–48
caller identification (ID) systems, 49
call volume, 8, 47
Cancer Care, Inc., 95
Cancer Information Service, 95
Cancer Institute of New Jersey, telephone triage policy at, 207–211
candidiasis, 118, 185
capecitabine, 137, 185
catheters, 89, 127, 197–199, 218
cellulitis, 185
central venous catheter, 197–199
certification, 52
check-off sheets, 22, 47
chemotherapy
    constipation from, 83
    diarrhea from, 97
    esophagitis from, 117
    flu-like symptoms from, 133
    hair loss from, 57–58
    hand-foot syndrome from, 137
    headache from, 141
    hematuria from, 145
    hemorrhagic cystitis from, 101
    mucositis from, 159
    myalgia/arthralgia from, 163, 165
    nausea/vomiting from, 167
    neutropenia from, 125–126
    pain from, 171
    peripheral neuropathy from, 175
    rash from, 185
    taste alterations from, 193
    xerostomia from, 201
chicken pox, 185
children, telenursing communication with, 49–50
chlorambucil, 185
chlorpromazine, 150
chronic cough, 87

chronic fatigue syndrome, 163
cisplatinum, 189
clerical employees, calls handled by, 32–33, 43
clinical competencies, of telephone triage nurses, 51–52
clonazepam, 68
coffee-ground-appearing material, in emesis, 168
College of Registered Nurses of Nova Scotia, 52
communication model, for telephone triage, 19
competencies, of telephone triage nurses, 51–52
complete blood count (CBC), 125
Complex Decongestive Therapy, 154
complex partial seizures, 189–191
compliance. See patient compliance
confidentiality, 28–29, 48–49
confirmation phase, of telephone triage, 19
confusion. See consciousness, change in level of
consciousness, change in level of, 79–81, 106, 110, 114, 118, 127, 142, 168–169, 190
constipation, 83–85
consultative calls, 31
continuing education, of telephone triage nurses, 51–52
contraceptives, 181, 191
cost reductions, from telenursing, 10
cough, 25, 87–88, 113, 127, 134
COX-2 inhibitors, 97
cultural differences, and telenursing, 50
Cushing's disease, 93
cyanosis, 113
cyclophosphamide, 101, 145, 185
cyclosporine, 189
cytarabine, 185, 201
cytomegalovirus syndrome, 163

D

data collection phase, of telephone triage, 19
deep venous thrombosis (DVT), 89–91
dehydration, 83, 98, 100, 126, 130, 160, 179
dengue fever, 163

Department of Health and Human Services, 95
depression/depressed mood, 69, 93–95, 121
dermatitis, 185
dermatomyositis, 185
dexamethasone, 165
diabetes mellitus, 79, 93, 106, 129, 133, 175, 186, 193
diagnosis, nursing vs. medical, 40
diarrhea, 83, 97–100
diazepam, 68
dietary changes
    constipation from, 83–84
    diarrhea from, 97–98
dietary fiber, 84–85
dietary guidelines. See also nutritional plan of care
    for anorexia, 64
    for ascites, 72
    for constipation, 84
    for diarrhea, 99
    for nausea/vomiting, 168
    for taste alterations, 194
dietary supplements, 64
diphenhydramine, 68, 138
disposition phase, of telephone triage, 19
diuretics, 97, 121, 201
dizziness, 105–106
    from anorexia, 63
    with diarrhea, 99
    with fatigue, 122
    with hematuria, 146
    with vomiting, 168
docetaxel, 163
documentation
    sample forms for, 212–216
    of telephone calls, 22, 26, 33, 45, 47
dopaminergic antagonists, 68
doxorubicin, 117, 137, 185, 201
dry mouth, 159, 193, 201–203
DVT. See deep venous thrombosis
dysphagia, 109–111, 117, 126, 193
dyspnea, 73, 113–115, 130
    with cough, 87–88, 113
    with hiccups, 149
    with menopausal symptoms, 155
    with rash, 186
dysuria, 101–102

E

edema, 153, 160
education, of telephone triage nurses, 51–52
elderly, telenursing communication with, 50–51
emergency departments (EDs)
    medical triage performed in, 7
    reasons for telephone calls to, 11
    telephone triage in, 11, 38
Emergency Nurses Association (ENA), 38
emergent causes, of headache, 141
emesis
    blood appearing in, 168
    brown/yellow/green, 84–85
    coffee-ground, 168
emollients, 138, 182
ENA. See Emergency Nurses Association
Ensure® supplement, 64
epidermal growth factor receptors, 185
epilepsy, 189–191
erythema multiforme, 185
erythema nodosum, 185
esophagitis, 109, 117–119
estrogen, 155
etoposide, 189
Eucerin®, 182
evaluation phase, of telephone triage, 13, 18, 42

F

fatigue, 121–123, 134
feeding tubes, 110–111, 117
feeling, loss of, 175–176
fever
    with neutropenia, 71, 102, 110, 118, 122, 125–127, 133, 146, 160, 168, 202
    without neutropenia, 101, 106, 129–131, 134, 146, 164, 186
fibromyalgia, 163
5-fluorouracil (5-FU), 97, 117, 185, 201
fluid accumulation, in peritoneal cavity, 71–73
flu-like symptoms, 102, 129, 133–134, 141–142
flurazepam, 68
flushing, of catheters, 199

follow-up calls, 26, 31–32, 35, 48
food, aversion to, 63–65
frequent callers, 26–27, 51
frontal (sinus) headaches, 141–142

G

gastrointestinal bleeding, 75, 106
gastrointestinal tubes, 110–111, 117
generalized seizures, 189–192
glomerulonephritis, 145
glossitis, 194
grand mal seizures, 189–192
growth factors, 163, 165
guidelines, for telephone triage, 12–13,
        21–23, 40–41, 46–47
    definition of, 21
    sample, 207–211
Guillain-Barré syndrome, 175

H

hair loss, 57–59
haloperidol, 68, 150
hand-foot syndrome, 137–139, 187
headache, 134, 141–143
    with fever, 130
    from infusions, 198
    with menopausal symptoms, 155
    with rash, 186
    with seizure, 190
hydroxyzine, 68
hyperesthesia head trauma, 142, 168,
        190
health advice, as part of telenursing, 5
health information, as part of
        telenursing, 5
health maintenance organizations, 6, 17
hematemesis, 75
hematopoietic growth factors, 163, 165
hematuria, 75, 102, 145–147
hemiparesis, 105–106
hemoptysis, 114
hemorrhagic cystitis, 101
herpes simplex, 185
herpes zoster, 185–186
hiccups, 149–150
high-grade fever, definition of, 129
HIPAA Privacy Rule, 48–49
HIV, 163
HMOs, 6, 17

hold, placing caller on, 26
Homan's sign, 90
hot flashes, 156, 186
hypocalcemia, 83
hypokalemia, 83
hyposalivation. See xerostomia
hypothyroidism, 93

I

ibuprofen, 165, 172
identity verification, 28, 49
ifosfamide, 101, 145, 189
imipenem, 189
immunotoxin, 165
impetigo, 185
implanted port, 197–199
implementation phase, of telephone
        triage, 13, 18, 42
infection
    dyspnea from, 114
    with mucositis, 159
    myalgia/arthralgia from, 163
    with neutropenia, 125–126
    rash from, 185–186
inpatient setting, vs. outpatient, 1, 10
insect bite, 164–165
insomnia, 157
Institute of Medicine (IOM), 22
insulin, 189
interferon, 141, 163, 165, 185
interleukin, 97, 145, 163, 165
interstate telenursing, legal issues
        concerning, 37, 39–40, 40t
interviewing skills, 27–29
intrathecal therapy, headache from, 141
IOM. See Institute of Medicine
irinotecan, 97
itch, 181–183, 187
IV therapy, phlebitis from, 179

J

JCAHO. See Joint Commission on
        Accreditation of Health Care
        Organizations
job descriptions, scope of practice
        outlined in, 43, 45
Joint Commission on Accreditation of
        Health Care Organizations
        (JCAHO), 38

jugular venous distention, during cough, 87, 114

K

kidney stones, 145

L

language barriers, in telenursing, 50
laxatives, 84, 97
legal issues, 32, 49–52
    of confidentiality, 48–49
    of liability, 43–48
    on nursing practice, 38–43, 40t
    and physician-patient communica-
        tion, 9
    on standards of care, 37–38
legal standards, 37
leg, severe pain in, 90, 155
leuprolide acetate, 145
levofloxacin, 189
liability, 43–45
    strategies to minimize, 45–48
licensure, of nurses, and telephone
        triage, 32, 37, 39–40, 40t, 43
lorazepam, 68
lotions, 138, 182
low-grade fever, definition of, 129
Lubriderm® lotion, 182
lupus, 185
Lyme disease, 163, 185
lymphedema, 153–154

M

malpractice, 9, 44
managed care, 6
Marinol® appetite stimulant, 64
measles, 185
mechlorethamine, 185
medical assistants, 43
medical triage, definition of, 6–7
medications
    causing anxiety/restlessness, 68
    causing constipation, 83
    causing depression, 93
    causing diarrhea, 97
    causing fatigue, 121
    causing headache, 141
    causing itching, 181
    causing seizures, 189
    causing xerostomia, 201
Megace® appetite stimulant, 64
Mehrabian Communication Model, 26
melena, 75
melphalan, 185
menopausal symptoms, 155–157
messages, leaving of, 28, 33–34, 49
methotrexate, 185, 201
methylphenidate, 68
metoclopramide, 68, 150
minors, telenursing communication
        with, 49–50
mouth rinses, 119, 161, 203
mucositis, 159–161, 202
muscle aches, generalized, 163–166
muscle relaxants, constipation from, 83
mutual recognition model, for interstate
        telenursing, 39–40, 40t
myalgia, 134, 163–166
myocardial infarction, 93

N

National Alliance for the Mentally Ill,
    95
National Certification Corporation, 52
National Committee for Quality
    Assurance (NCQA), 38
National Council of State Boards of
    Nursing (NCSBN), 5, 7, 39, 40t
National Depressive and Manic
    Depressive Association, 95
National Foundation for Depressive
    Illness, 95
National Mental Health Association, 95
nausea/vomiting, 167–169
    from ascites, 72
    with constipation, 84
    with dizziness, 105–106
NCSBN. See National Council of State
    Boards of Nursing
negligence, 44. See also liability
neutropenia, fever with, 71, 102, 110,
    118, 122, 125–127, 133, 146,
    160, 168, 202
Nevada State Board of Nursing,
    telenursing position statements
    on, 41, 43
nifedipine, 150
Nivea® lotion, 182

nocturia, 102
noncompliance. *See* patient compliance
nonemergent causes, of headache, 141
nonverbal messages, in communication, 26
nonvertiginous dizziness, 105
numbness, 175–176
Nurse Licensure Compact, 39–40, 40*t*
nursing diagnosis, legal definition of, 42
nursing practice
   legal issues concerning, 38–43
   scope of, 42–43
   telenursing classified as, 7, 39
nursing process, used in telephone triage, 12–13, 17–18, 42–43
Nursing Spectrum (communications company), 1
nursing standards, 37–38
nutritional plan of care. *See also* dietary guidelines
   for dysphagia, 110
   for esophagitis, 118
   for xerostomia, 202
nutritional supplements, 64

O

Occupational Safety and Health Administration (OSHA), 38
odynophagia, 117
OLD CART assessment, for telephone triage, 18–19
open-ended questions, use of, 25, 27, 51
opioids, 181, 201
oral hygiene, 119, 126, 161, 203
orientation, of telephone triage nurses, 51
orthostatic hypotension, 63
OSHA. *See* Occupational Safety and Health Administration
outpatient setting, vs. inpatient, 1, 10

P

paclitaxel, 163
pain, 171–173
pain diary, 172
palmar-plantar erythrodysesthesia, 137–139, 187
paraneoplastic syndromes, 163

paresthesia, 175–177, 186
partial seizures, 189–192
passwords, use of, 28, 49
pathologic cough, 87
patient compliance, 10, 35
patient confidentiality, 28–29, 48–49
patient satisfaction, 10, 47
pegylated liposomal doxorubicin, 137
Pennsylvania, nursing diagnosis defined in, 42
pericardial effusion, 113
peripherally inserted central catheter (PICC), 197–199
peripheral neuropathy, 175–177
peritoneal cavity, fluid accumulation in, 71–73
personal standards, 37
petechia, 75
petit mal seizures, 189, 191
phenothiazines, 68
phenytoin, 150
phlebitis, 179–180
photophobia/photosensitivity, 130, 142
phrenic nerve block, 150
planning phase, during telephone triage, 12–13, 18, 42
platelets, decreased number of, 75
PLISSIT Model, for discussing sexual concerns, 62
policies/procedures, 13, 45–46, 207–211. *See also* guidelines, for telephone triage
position sense, loss of, 175
P, Q, R, S, T, and T system, for telephone triage, 18
prednisone, 165
primary lymphedema, 153
privacy issues, 28–29, 48–49
problem-oriented system, for telephone triage, 18
process standards, 38
prochlorperazine, 68
professional standards/organizations, 38
projectile vomiting, 168–169
promethazine, 68
prostatitis, 101
ProSure® supplement, 64
protocols, for telephone triage, 12–13, 21–23, 40–41, 46–47
   definition of, 21
   sample, 207–211

proton-pump inhibitors, 117, 119
pruritus, 181–183, 187
psychostimulants, 68
pump, ambulatory, 199, 218

Q

quality assurance programs, 48, 217–218

R

radiation therapy
   diarrhea from, 97
   dysphagia from, 109
   hair loss from, 58
   headache from, 141
   hematuria from, 145
   mucositis from, 159
   nausea/vomiting from, 167
   neutropenia from, 125
   pain from, 171
   prostatitis from, 101
   rash from, 185
   taste alterations from, 193
   xerostomia from, 201
rash, 137, 181–183, 185–188
rectal bleeding, 84, 99
red streaks
   with lymphedema, 153
   with phlebitis, 179–180
   with venous access device, 197–198
referral, to other services, 45, 47
regulatory standards/agencies, 38
repeat callers, 26–27, 51
restating, during telephone communication, 27
retrobulbar headaches, 141–142
rotation, of telephone triage duty, 32
rubella, 185

S

saliva decrease. *See* xerostomia
satisfaction. *See* patient satisfaction
scabies, 182, 185
screening of calls, by clerical employees, 32–33
secondary lymphedema, 153
seizures, 80, 189–192
sexuality, alterations in, 61–62, 94

Sexuality and Cancer, 62
shortness of breath, 73, 113–115, 130
   with cough, 87–88, 113
   with hiccups, 149
   with menopausal symptoms, 155
SIADH (syndrome of inappropriate antidiuretic hormone secretion), 141
silicone implant syndrome, 163
simethicone, 150
simple partial seizures, 189–191
sinus headaches, 141
skin changes, 137–139, 181–183, 185–188
socioeconomic differences, and telenursing, 50
sorbitol medications, 97
standards of care, 37–38
state boards of nursing, 38–42
state lines, telenursing across, legal issues concerning, 37, 39–40, 40*t*
states' rights amendment, 39
steroids, 68, 129, 163, 165
Stevens-Johnson syndrome, 186
stomatitis, 194
stool softeners, 84
streaks/streaking. *See* red streaks
stridor, 87, 186
structural standards, 38
suicidal ideation, 93–94, 156
support groups, 95
surveillance calls, 32
swallowing, difficulty in, 109–111, 117, 126, 193
syncope, 142
syndrome of inappropriate antidiuretic hormone secretion (SIADH), 141

T

tacrolimus, 189
taste alterations, 193–195
taxanes, 163, 165, 175
Telecommunications Device for the Deaf (TDD), 50
Telehealth Nursing Practice Administration and Practice Standards (AAACN), 52
telemedicine, definition of, 5–6

telephone mediated care, telephone triage described as, 8
"Telephone Medical Advice Services" (California law), 41
Telephone Nursing Practice Certification, 52
telephone triage/telenursing
    cost reductions resulting from, 10
    definition of, 5, 7–8
    general tips on performing, 25–29
    guidelines/protocols for, 12–13, 21–23, 40–41, 46–47, 207–211
    history of, 6
    legal concerns of, 37–53
    models of, 17–20
    as nursing practice, 7, 39
    nursing process used in, 12–13, 17–18, 42–43
temazepam, 68
temperature sensation, loss of, 175
Tenth Amendment, 39
thiotepa, 185
thrombocytopenia, 75–77, 142
thrombocytopenic purpura, 185
thrombus, 89–91
tick bite, 164–165
time spent on calls, optimum, 34–35, 51
tingling, 175–176
tonic-clonic seizures, 189–192
tranquilizers, constipation from, 83
translator services, 50
triage, definition of, 6–7. See also telephone triage/telenursing
tunneled central venous catheter, 197–199

U

Udderly Smooth® cream, 138
unconsciousness, 79
urinary retention, 101

urinary tract infection, 101, 145
urination, difficulty/pain with, 101–102, 127, 130, 146
urine changes. See also hematuria
    with ascites, 73
    with diarrhea, 99

V

vaginal bleeding, 155
vaginal dryness, 156
valproic acid, 150
vasculitis, 163
vein, inflammation of. See phlebitis
venous access devices, problems with, 89, 127, 197–199, 218
vertiginous dizziness/vertigo, 105
vibratory sense, loss of, 175
vinblastine, 201
vinca alkaloids, 175
vincristine, 201
virus/viral symptoms, 114, 167, 187
visual changes, 142, 169, 190
vitamin B_6, 176
voice mail, 28, 33–34, 49
vomiting. See emesis; nausea/vomiting

W

weight gain, from ascites, 72
weight loss
    from anorexia, 63–65
    from depression, 94
    from diarrhea, 98
    from dysphagia, 109
    from esophagitis, 117
    with taste alterations, 193–194
wheezing, 87, 113–114, 130, 186

X

xerostomia, 159, 193, 201–203